Fertility Mastery Guide

Taking charge of your Fertility

Unlocking the Pathways to Fertility: A Comprehensive Guide to Mastering Your Reproductive Health

Thomas T. Stewart

Table Contents

CONTENT 1.
INTRODUCTION

<u>Introduction: Opening the Pathways to Fruitfulness Mastery</u>

Leaving on the striking excursion towards life as a parent is a profoundly private and extraordinary experience. The "Ripeness Dominance Guide" isn't simply an aide; it's your unflinching buddy through the unpredictable labyrinth of richness improvement. Whether you're making your most memorable strides or have been exploring this street for some time, this guide is intended to engage you with information that rises above the customary.

Dive into a reality where science and soul interlace, where comprehensive methodologies fit with state of the art clinical experiences. Investigate the ensemble of sustenance, way of life, and profound prosperity that organizes your conceptive wellbeing. This guide is definitely not a simple assortment of realities - it's an organized story of trust, versatility, and strengthening.

Plan to reveal the insider facts of richness following, to graph your special course through the floods of ovulation. Find how the climate you possess can be finely tuned to make a shelter for richness to thrive. What's more, as you set out on this journey, you'll find accounts of people who've prevailed over misfortune, lighting the way with their triumphs.

The way to richness authority is all around as different as the people who track it, and this guide is your compass, directing you toward your own form of progress. Lock in, in light of the fact that you're going to leave on an undertaking that blends shrewdness with amazement, science with otherworldliness, and planning with unadulterated, unrestrained chance. Your process starts here.

In the peaceful minutes when dreams entwine with the real world, the craving for life as a parent flourishes, developing into an intense excursion that reshapes lives. Welcome to an aide that enlightens this way more than ever - the "Fruitfulness Dominance Guide."

Envision an embroidery woven from the strings of state of the art science, old insight, and the faithful soul of those who've set out on this odyssey. With each turn of the page, you're welcome to step into a reality where each detail matters, every choice conveys weight, and every decision leads you nearer to the support of plausibility.

Here, you'll investigate the significant effect of nourishment, as your body turns into a material where richness is supported. Figure out what the mood of your life means for the orchestra of chemicals that get into the rhythm of origination. Past the physical, dive into the domains of close to home prosperity, where the scene of trust and steadiness comes to fruition.

Feel the beat of ripeness following, a window into your body's mood, a guide to your most prolific days. Find the speculative chemistry of establishing a ripeness accommodating climate, where each breath you take, each corner you contact, contrive to make an ideal safe-haven for life to thrive.

However, this guide is more than statistical data points; it's a journey through stories - stories of those who've strolled this way, drawing signs of boldness and winning. These accounts are the heavenly body that guides you through unsure evenings, helping you that the stars to remember probability sparkle splendidly, even in the haziest skies.

Thus, open these pages with a heart brimming with expectation and a psyche prepared to retain the complexities of fruitfulness dominance. This is your door to an existence where science and yearning meet, where information turns into a lamp enlightening the way to life as a parent. As you step into this domain of revelation, recall that every section holds the way to opening the potential inside you. Your process starts now.

Figuring out the Intricacies of Richness: Divulging Nature's Complicated Design

Envision looking at an embroidery woven from the strings of science, hereditary qualities, and the sensitive interchange of chemicals - this is the dazzling vista that "Figuring out the Intricacies of Ripeness" discloses before you. In this section, we set out on an undertaking to disentangle the mystery that is fruitfulness, investigating its layers with the interest

of a researcher and the marvel of a
traveler.

At its center, ripeness is an ensemble of
complexities that agreeably meets to
make life. Jump into the domain of
regenerative science, where the
complicated dance of chemicals
coordinates the ascent and fall of
ovulation, winding around a mood that
reverberations through time.
Comprehend what the equilibrium of
these compound couriers means for the
fragile harmony among fruitfulness and
barrenness, laying out a picture of
probability with each cycle.

Yet, richness isn't exclusively the domain
of chemicals; it's the combination of
hereditary qualities, climate, and way of
life. Dig into the hereditary embroidered
artwork that shapes ripeness,
investigating what individual varieties

can mean for the capacity to consider. Adventure further into the universe of epigenetics, where the decisions can make a permanent imprint on people in the future.

As you explore this section, you'll experience the intricacy of timing - the fragile dance of synchronizing ovulation, treatment, and implantation. Reveal the science behind fruitfulness following techniques, from basal internal heat level to cervical bodily fluid investigation, every strategy offering a novel window into your body's rhythms.

Past the science, embrace the close to home aspect that goes with the excursion. Fruitfulness' intricacies stretch out to the significant close to home scene of trust, vulnerability, and strength. Gain from the narratives of those who've endured the hardships, arising more grounded not set in stone on the opposite side.

In this part, we dare to demystify the many-sided puzzle of fruitfulness, piece by piece, idea by idea. As you submerge yourself in the realm of natural wonders, hereditary disclosures, and the significant feelings that string through this embroidery, you'll find yourself outfitted with freshly discovered experiences. Allow this excursion to be a demonstration of the mind blowing orchestra of life, where understanding the intricacies of fruitfulness turns into an extension interfacing you to the significant excellence of creation itself.

Figuring out the Excursion to Ripeness Dominance: Exploring the Profundities of Desire

Underneath the outer layer of each and every yearning, a vast expanse of intricacy anticipates - and your journey for richness dominance is no special case. Welcome to a part that fills in as both endlessly compass, diagramming the course through unfamiliar waters.

Leaving on this excursion isn't simply about considering a youngster; it's tied in with embracing the significant orchestra of life, where science meets feeling, science meets otherworldliness, and dreams change into the real world. Envision yourself at the edge of understanding, prepared to assimilate the significant bits of knowledge that lie ahead.

In these pages, you'll unwind the conundrum of richness, plunging profound into the multifaceted components that shape origination. From the fragile dance of chemicals to the transaction of hereditary qualities and way of life, each piece of the riddle adds to the work of art that is your regenerative wellbeing.

However, this excursion isn't one-layered - it's embroidery woven with strings of trust and flexibility. Investigate the close to home landscape, where the longing for life as a parent crashes into the floods of vulnerability. Find the strength inside you, the ability to deal with difficulties directly, and the capacity to change mishaps into venturing stones.

The excursion to richness authority is about more than information; it's about point of view. It's tied in with looking at the skyline of probability and understanding that each step carries you more like an objective that is extraordinarily yours. As you submerge yourself in this section, imagine the woven artwork of your own process coming to fruition, and let the disclosures guide you toward the authority you look for.

CONTENT. 2 2. Foundation of Fertility

Underpinning of Fruitfulness: Divulging the Outline of Possibility

Welcome to the bedrock of your excursion - the part that reveals the establishment whereupon the ensemble of life is created. " Underpinning of Ripeness" isn't simply an assortment of realities; a disclosure of the outline shapes your regenerative predetermination.

Envision looking into the mind boggling design of your DNA, where the dance of hereditary qualities and epigenetics coordinates the potential forever. In this part, we venture into the domains of acquired qualities, investigating the strings that connect ages and the unobtrusive murmurs of qualities that convey the expectations representing things to come.

Be that as it may, hereditary qualities are simply the introduction; a way of life arises as a focal hero. Investigate the halls of sustenance, where the sustenance you give your body turns into the material whereupon ripeness paints its magnum opus. Dig into the crossing point of diet and regenerative wellbeing, figuring out how certain supplements become the structure blocks of ripeness and how way of life decisions can either sustain or upset the sensitive harmony.

As we explore further, the orchestra reaches out to the climate around you. Reveal the secret effect of ordinary components - from contaminations to stretch - on the unpredictable instruments of origination. This part enables you to organize a richness accommodating climate, where the actual setting turns into a supporting person in your excursion.

Get ready to be submerged in the study of hormonal equilibrium, where the complexities of insulin, thyroid chemicals, and regenerative chemicals entwine. Find how way of life and hereditary qualities team up to impact chemical levels, affecting fruitfulness as well as your general prosperity.

The "Groundwork of Ripeness" is where the unique pieces fit together, shaping an extensive image of the stuff to make life.

A section engages you with information and highlights the job you play in molding your contraceptive predetermination. As you explore through these pages, recollect that understanding the establishment is the way to building the way toward ripeness dominance.

Investigating the Study of Propagation: Divulging the Complexities of Life's Genesis

Plan to leave on a journey through the actual substance of presence - the part "Investigating the Study of Multiplication" welcomes you to look into the complexities of life's most significant secret. With the interest of a pilgrim and the miracle of a researcher, we venture through the embroidery of natural wonders that shape the supernatural occurrence of birth.

Envision remains at the edge of creation, where the combination of gametes turns into the flash that lights life. In this section, we take apart the phases of proliferation, from the stunning expressive dance of meiosis - where chromosomes dance and trade hereditary data - to the union of egg and sperm in an orchestra of cell predetermination.

However, the science doesn't stop at origination; it reaches out to the great excursion of embryogenesis. Navigate the scene where a solitary cell increases into a mind boggling organic entity, every division a stroke of imaginative accuracy. Unwind the tales composed inside the qualities, as they guide the diagram of advancement, directing everything from the shade of eyes to the mood of pulses.

As we investigate further, uncover the unique powers behind the change of a prepared egg into an undeveloped organism, and in the long run, a hatchling. From the coordination of organ development to the multifaceted dance of chemicals that supports pregnancy, each part of this story is a disclosure of nature's brightness.

However, the science is nevertheless a string woven into the embroidery. Winding through this part are the accounts of strength - the stories of those who've resisted chances and won over moves on their excursion to being a parent. These accounts advise us that science, while stunning, is only one aspect of the excursion; boldness and trust are its undaunted friends.

"Investigating the Study of Generation" isn't simply a section; it's an entry into the actual heart of life's beginning. Through these pages, the secret turns into a guide, and the intricacies change into disclosures. Plan to be enraptured, for the excursion will undoubtedly leave you in wonderment of the mind boggling dance that brings about presence itself.

Factors Influencing Richness: Hereditary qualities, Way of life, and Environment

Leave on an excursion through the embroidery of ripeness, where the strings of hereditary qualities, way of life, and climate entwine to shape the magnum opus of origination. In this part, we plunge into the unpredictable trap of impacts that decide your richness process

- a journey that blends science with your special hereditary code, the decisions, and the world that encompasses you.

Envision your hereditary qualities as the compass, directing the course of your fruitfulness journey. Here, we open the mysteries held inside your DNA, finding how acquired qualities impact conceptive results. From the outline of egg and sperm to the mosaic of hereditary varieties, you'll uncover the fingerprints of previous eras and future, all woven into the texture of fruitfulness.

Way of life arises as another hero, a co-creator of your richness story. Investigate the effect of diet, exercise, and weight on your regenerative wellbeing. As you venture through the sections of nourishment, actual work, and stress the board, you'll uncover the power you hold to shape your body's preparation for origination.

The material of ripeness stretches out past your being; it incorporates the climate that wraps you. Dig into the domain of ecological elements - from contaminations to radiation - that can impact regenerative wellbeing. Outfitted with this information, you can organize a space that sustains ripeness, changing your environmental factors into a safe-haven for origination.

As you navigate this section, recollect that you're not just an inactive member; you're an engaged hero in your ripeness story. By grasping the complicated dance of hereditary qualities, way of life, and climate, you're prepared to settle on decisions that blend with your yearnings. Every disclosure is a stepping stone on the way to richness dominance, a way

where information enables you to
co-make the excursion you imagine.

What Are The Factors Affecting Fertility: Genetics, Lifestyle, and Environment

Factors influencing ripeness are perplexing and diverse, including a blend of hereditary, way of life, and ecological components. This is an outline of the way each variable can affect richness:

1. Genetics:
Hereditary elements assume a critical part in ripeness. Acquired attributes and hereditary varieties can impact conceptive results. Hereditary circumstances, chromosomal irregularities, and quality

transformations can affect richness in all kinds of people. Furthermore, certain hereditary variables can influence the planning of menopause, ovarian hold, and weakness to conditions like polycystic ovary disorder (PCOS) and endometriosis.

2. Lifestyle:
Way of life decisions can significantly affect fruitfulness. These decisions include:

- Diet: Wholesome factors, for example, body weight, admission of specific supplements (like folate, zinc, and cell reinforcements), and exorbitant caffeine or liquor utilization can influence ripeness.
- Exercise:Both inadequate and unnecessary active work can upset hormonal equilibrium and periods,

possibly influencing ovulation and fruitfulness.

- Smoking: Smoking is connected to diminished fruitfulness in all kinds of people, influencing sperm quality, ovarian capability, and undeveloped organism implantation.
- Liquor and Medication Use: Over the top liquor utilization and sporting medication use can obstruct hormonal equilibrium and contraceptive capability.
- Stress: Persistent pressure can influence chemical creation and upset periods, possibly influencing ovulation and richness.

3. Environment:
Natural variables can impact ripeness through openness to poisons, contaminations, and radiation. These elements include:

- Endocrine Disruptors: Synthetic substances tracked down in certain plastics, pesticides, and individual consideration items can mirror chemicals and disrupt the endocrine framework, possibly influencing fruitfulness.
- Pollution: Air contamination and openness to ecological poisons can influence sperm quality and conceptive wellbeing.
- Radiation: Elevated degrees of radiation openness, for example, from specific operations or word related perils, can influence regenerative cells and richness.

It's essential to take note that every individual's fruitfulness process is remarkable. While these elements can influence fruitfulness, the level of effect fluctuates from one individual to another. Going with informed decisions about way of life, looking for clinical counsel when required, and establishing a strong climate can add to streamlining richness. Assuming ripeness challenges emerge, talking with medical services experts representing considerable authority in conceptual wellbeing can give direction and customized arrangements.

Conclusion: Exploring the Ternion of Fruitfulness Influences

As we finish up our investigation into the perplexing embroidery of richness, it's obvious that the excursion to origination is an orchestra made out of three amicable components: hereditary qualities, way of life, and climate. Each variable contributes its remarkable notes to the tune, making a piece that is however mind boggling as it could be entrancing.

Hereditary qualities, the quiet orchestrator, winds around the strings of previous eras and future into the texture of richness. It lays out a representation of acquired characteristics and expected difficulties, helping us to remember the multifaceted dance between our natural cosmetics and the pathways to life as a parent.

Way of life, the guide of decision, engages us to play a functioning job in our richness story. Through cognizant choices about sustenance, work out, stress the executives, and that's only the tip of the iceberg, we employ the ability to shape the cadence of our regenerative wellbeing. This section's disclosures guide us toward making a way of life that reverberates with our desires.

Climate, the scenery of our excursion, makes way for ripeness to thrive or flounder. From contaminations to radiation, our environmental factors can possibly affect our conceptive wellbeing. Outfitted with information, we have the devices to change our current circumstance into a sustaining safe-haven for origination.

In this orchestra of impacts, we are not detached audience members; we are dynamic members, writers of our own ripeness account. Equipped with understanding, we can settle on informed choices that guide us toward ripeness authority. Whether the excursion is smooth or experiences difficulties, the information we've acquired enables us to explore with certainty and flexibility.

As you leave on your way ahead, recollect that hereditary qualities, way of life, and climate are the notes that mix into a remarkable tune, a song that resounds with the rhythms of your heart and the fantasies in your eyes. May your process be directed by the orchestra of intelligence and trust, as you draw nearer to the crescendo of life as a parent, where each note is a demonstration of the force of understanding and strengthening.

Exploring Fruitfulness' Intersection: Enabling Solutions

As we explore the junction of hereditary qualities, way of life, and climate with regards to fruitfulness, the excursion turns into an embroidery of strengthening and potential outcomes.

Here, we disclose arrangements that offer a compass for those looking to improve their ripeness process:

1. Genetics:
While we can't adjust our hereditary diagram, we can use progressions in regenerative medication to alleviate hereditary difficulties. Hereditary advising and assumption testing give experiences into possible dangers, assisting people with coming to informed conclusions about family arranging. Helped conceptive innovations, similar to preimplantation hereditary testing, take into consideration the choice of incipient organisms with less hereditary irregularities.

2. Lifestyle:
Strengthening lies in our decisions consistently. Embrace a decent eating regimen wealthy in fruitfulness helping

supplements, keep a solid weight, and take part in customary actual work. Focus on pressure decreases through rehearsals like yoga, reflection, and care. Stop smoking and breaking point liquor admission to establish a climate that upholds hormonal equilibrium and regenerative wellbeing.

3. Environment:
Tackle the force of cognizant living to establish a climate that welcomes fruitfulnesses. Select natural and poison free items to diminish openness to endocrine disruptors. Limit openness to contamination by picking clean air courses while practicing and staying away from regions with weighty traffic. Focus on wellbeing while going through operations including radiation, and discuss straightforwardly with medical care experts about your fruitfulness concerns.

4. Looking for Proficient Guidance:
While exploring the intricacies of
richness, it is vital to look for master
direction. Talking with a contraceptive
endocrinologist, fruitfulness subject
matter expert, or hereditary instructor
can give customized experiences and
proposals. They can assist with tending
to explicit hereditary worries, offer
fruitfulness evaluations, and guide you
toward customized methodologies to
enhance your possibilities of origination.

5. Support and Resilience:
Perceive that the ripeness excursion can
genuinely challenge. Encircle yourself
with an encouraging group of people of
friends and family, companions, and
richness support gatherings. Sharing
encounters and gaining from others
who've confronted comparable

difficulties can give close to home strength and versatility.

In the combination of hereditary qualities, way of life, and climate, arrangements arise as strings that tight spot the woven artwork of richness together. Embrace the strengthening that information brings, and let these arrangements be your partners as you set out on your excursion toward life as a parent. Recollect that while difficulties might emerge, the ensemble of arrangements guides you toward the agreeable song of probability, where dreams find their reverberation and expectations are changed into real factors.

CONTENT. 3.Nutrition and Fertility

Sustenance and Fruitfulness: Feeding the Way to Parenthood

In the complex dance of richness, nourishment arises as a director that organizes the cadence of regenerative wellbeing. This part uncovers the significant effect of what you consume - on your general prosperity, however on the complex systems that support origination. As we venture through the domains of supplements, balance, and careful eating, you'll find that the food you pick is a powerful mixture that can either blend or disturb the ensemble of richness.

Envision your body as a material, painted stroke by stroke with the shades of supplements. In this section, we investigate the structure blocks of richness, from folate and zinc to omega-3 unsaturated fats and cell reinforcements. Every supplement assumes an exceptional part in supporting regenerative capability, impacting all that from egg quality to chemical equilibrium.

Adjusting the scales is one more essential component of the fruitfulness condition. The fragile interaction between body weight and ripeness is a point of convergence, as the two limits - underweight and overweight - can upset hormonal congruity and influence ovulation. With bits of knowledge into the association between Weight Record

(BMI) and contraceptive wellbeing, you'll figure out how to explore the way of harmony.

Past the physical, the mental parts of sustenance become the overwhelming focus. Find the connection among stress and eating designs, as well as systems to develop careful eating. By sustaining your body with goal and mindfulness, you establish a climate that upholds your general wellbeing as well as your fruitfulness process.

As you venture through this part, recall that nourishment isn't simply food; an impetus fills the multifaceted hardware of origination. Each feast is a chance to put resources into your ripeness, to give your body the assets it necessities to make life. Thus, relish the information you uncover here, and let it guide your decisions as you sustain the way to life as a parent, each chomp in turn.

Sustaining Your Direction to Origination: Dietary Rules for Fertility

Leaving on the excursion to being a parent is a significant undertaking, and one of the most enabling devices available to you is the food you decide to sustain your body. This section is your manual for figuring out the harmonious connection among nourishment and ripeness - a relationship that can essentially influence your possibilities of origination.

1. Embrace Supplement Rich Foods: Consider your body a nursery that requires support. Choose an eating

routine wealthy in entire, natural food sources like organic products, vegetables, lean proteins, entire grains, nuts, and seeds. These supplement thick decisions give fundamental nutrients, minerals, and cancer prevention agents that help contraceptive wellbeing.

2. Focus on Folate and B Vitamins: Folate, a B-nutrient, assumes a critical part in the fetal turn of events. Guarantee your eating routine incorporates wellsprings of folate like mixed greens, vegetables, and strengthened grains. B nutrients, including B6 and B12, are likewise significant for chemical guidelines and ovulation.

3. Omega-3 Greasy Acids: These fundamental fats resemble the oil for your regenerative framework. Tracked down in greasy fish, pecans, flaxseeds, and chia seeds, omega-3

unsaturated fats support hormonal
equilibrium and egg quality.

4. Cell reinforcement Powerhouses:
Vivid foods grown from the ground are
your partners in the battle against
oxidative pressure. Berries, citrus natural
products, and mixed greens are wealthy
cancer prevention agents that shield your
eggs and sperm from harm.

5. Lean Protein Sources:
Incorporate lean protein sources like
poultry, fish, eggs, and plant-based
proteins. Protein is fundamental for
chemical creation and keeps up with
consistent glucose levels.

6. Complex Carbohydrates:
Pick entire grains like quinoa, earthy
colored rice, and oats. Complex starches
give supported energy and forestall quick

spikes in glucose, supporting hormonal equilibrium.

7. Oversee Sugar and Trans Fats:
Limit sweet food sources and drinks as well as trans fats tracked down in broiled and handled food varieties. High sugar consumption and trans fats can disturb chemical guidelines and fruitfulness.

8. Remain Hydrated:
Water is fundamental for general wellbeing, and remaining appropriately hydrated upholds the soundness of your cervical bodily fluid - an imperative part for sperm endurance and transportation.

9. Caffeine and Liquor Moderation:
While moderate caffeine utilization is by and large thought to be protected, unnecessary caffeine admission might obstruct origination. Limit liquor

utilization, as unreasonable drinking is related with diminished ripeness.

10. Keep a Solid Weight:
Take a stab at a sound BMI, as being either underweight or overweight can influence chemical creation and ovulation. Hold back nothing diet that upholds a feasible weight.

11. Look for Proficient Guidance:
Talk with an enlisted dietitian or medical care proficient who works in ripeness sustenance. They can give customized proposals in light of your singular requirements and clinical history.

Keep in mind, the excursion to origination is tied in with supporting your body as well as your fantasies. By embracing these dietary rules, you're making an establishment that upholds fruitfulness and encourages the chance of making life. Every dinner turns into a careful move toward being a parent, an approach to sustaining your direction to origination with each feeding tear you take.

Fundamental Supplements for Contraceptive Wellbeing: Feeding the Seeds of Life

Open the key to sustaining your ripeness with the strong elixirs of fundamental supplements. This section is an enrapturing venture through the culinary scene, where every supplement rich chomp turns into a bit nearer to making life. Envision yourself relishing the kinds of plausibility as we investigate the essential job that these supplements play in your contraceptive excursion.

1. Folate: The Gatekeeper of Growth
Meet folate, the overlooked yet truly
great individual of origination. Jump into
the universe of mixed greens, lentils, and
citrus organic products - all rich
wellsprings of this B-nutrient that
safeguards your child-to-be from brain
tube deformities and supports the
earliest transformative phases.

2. Omega-3 Unsaturated fats: The
Ensemble of Sustenance
Envision your body as an ensemble, and
omega-3 unsaturated fats as the amicable
notes that help hormonal equilibrium
and egg quality. Find the appeal of
wild-gotten salmon, chia seeds, and
pecans - nature's symphony for
conceptive wellbeing.

3. Iron: The Remedy of Energy
Disclose the mystery of iron's dance
through your veins. This mineral, tracked

down in lean meats, beans, and strengthened grains, conveys the oxygen that fills your conceptual framework. Feel the liveliness of expanded energy and essentialness that iron brings to your ripeness process.

4. Vitamin D: The Daylight Nutrient of Fertility
Lounge in the warm hug of vitamin D, the daylight supplement that upholds your bones as well as your regenerative wellbeing. Investigate its sources - from invigorated dairy to absorbing daylight - and embrace the essentialness it offers to your way to life as a parent.

5. Antioxidants: The Watchmen of the Ovum
Envision cell reinforcements as sentinels, protecting your valuable eggs from the desolates of time. Find the ensemble of variety in berries, chime peppers, and

mixed greens - each nibble an eruption of security against oxidative pressure that can influence richness.

6. Zinc: The Weaver of Hereditary Threads
Enter the domain of zinc, the fundamental mineral that winds around the texture of hereditary material. From helping egg quality to supporting sperm wellbeing, find this micronutrient in clams, pumpkin seeds, and lean meats, lighting the flash of life.

7. L-ascorbic acid: The Mixture of Immunity
Imagine L-ascorbic acid as a safeguard, shielding your contraceptive wellbeing from the attack of free revolutionaries. Submerge yourself in citrus organic products, chime peppers, and strawberries - each nibble a taste from

the wellspring of safe help and imperativeness.

8. B Nutrients: The Hormonal Harmony Envision B nutrients as the directors of hormonal congruity, coordinating ovulation and ripeness. Dive into sources like eggs, lean meats, and entire grains, as these B nutrients make the song out of contraceptive health.

With each supplement stuffed piece, you're supporting the seeds of life, creating an ensemble of sustenance that reverberates with the commitment of probability. These fundamental supplements become your partners, engaging your ripeness process with flavors that stir your taste buds as well as your fantasies of life as a parent.

CONTENT 4.Lifestyle Optimization

Way of life Streamlining: Chiseling Your Richness Canvas

Envision your life as a material, trusting that your strokes of expectation will shape the work of art of your fruitfulness process. In this section, we dive into the specialty of way of life improvement - a cycle that goes past daily practice to make an energetic embroidery of health that upgrades your contraceptive potential. Get ready to set out on an excursion where every decision you make turns into a brushstroke, winding around an account of strengthening and plausibility.

1. The Dance of Actual Activity:
Envision yourself traveling through existence with essentialness, as actual work turns into your accomplice in this dance of richness. Whether it's a lively walk, a yoga stream, or a dance class, each step upgrades blood flow, upholds hormonal equilibrium, and adds to a body that is prepared for origination.

2. Weight The board: Adjusting the Sizes of Wellness:
Envision your body as a scale, with balance as the way to regenerative congruity. Investigate the idea of Weight List (BMI) as an aide, understanding how keeping a solid weight can streamline ovulation and improve your possibilities of origination.

3. Stress: The Specialty of Reestablishing Balance:

Imagine pressure as a material of feelings, sitting tight for you to paint it with the shades of unwinding and quiet. Uncover the association among stress and ripeness, and find care, contemplation, and profound breathing as brushes that reestablish close to home balance and backing conceptive wellbeing.

4. Sleep: The Sweeping of Restoration:

Picture rest as a delicate cover that folds over you, sustaining your body as well as your fruitfulness goals. Figure out the complicated dance among rest and hormonal equilibrium, and figure out how to embrace solid rest propensities as a foundation of your fruitfulness process.

5. Restricting Poisons: Making a Ripeness Accommodating Environment:

Envision your environmental factors as a safe-haven, liberated from the hold of poisons that can disturb regenerative health. Investigate the force of cognizant decisions in day to day existence, from picking perfect, natural items to decreasing openness to ecological poisons that can affect richness.

6. Smoking and Liquor: Modifying the Way of life Canvas:
Picture your way of life material developing as you move back from hurtful propensities. Investigate the hindering effect of smoking and unnecessary liquor utilization on richness, and consider this part your range for making a smoke, moderate liquor way of life.

7. Correspondence and Association: Meshing Backing into Your Journey:

Envision correspondence as strings that tight spot your ripeness process to an organization of help. Interface with your accomplice, companions, family, and care groups to share encounters, trade counsel, and cultivate profound prosperity during this extraordinary section of life.

In this section, you're not simply finding out about ways of life enhancement - you're submerged during the time spent chiseling a rich life that resounds with essentialness and expectation. With each brushstroke of actual work, each demonstration of stress decrease, and each careful decision, you're making a show-stopper that fits with your goals. Welcome to the specialty of way of life streamlining, where your material turns into an impression of your commitment to supporting the seeds of life.

Stress The executives Procedures for Richness Improvement: Exploring Quiet Waters to Conception

In the multifaceted dance of richness, stress can be both an impressive foe and a conquerable test. This part unwinds the significant association among stress and regenerative wellbeing, offering a gold mine of procedures to explore the wild waters of pressure, and in doing as such, improve your ripeness process.

1. Mindfulness: Embracing the Present Moment
Envision yourself established in the present, liberated from the shackles of stresses over the past or tensions about what's in store. Care is your compass, directing you toward internal harmony

and close to home equilibrium. Through procedures like profound breathing, body sweeps, and reflection, you figure out how to tame the turbulent flows of pressure, sustaining a ripe climate inside.

2. Meditation: Developing Peacefulness Within

Imagine yourself in a quiet safe-haven, where the commotion of stress scatters into the serenity of your psyche. Reflection turns into your asylum, permitting you to separate from outer disarray and reconnect with your internal identity. As you cut out snapshots of tranquility, you're chiseling a shelter of harmony that reverberations in the musicality of your pulses.

3. Yoga: The Agreement of Body and Mind

Envision your body as an instrument, every yoga represents a note that plays as

one with your spirit. Yoga turns into your
tune of equilibrium, as the training draws
in your body, brain, and breath. With
each stretch and posture, you disentangle
pressure, freeing both body and soul
from the grip of pressure.

4. Exercise: Directing Pressure into
Movement
Picture pressure as energy flowing
through your veins, ready to be changed.
Practice turns into your course,
permitting you to channel pressure into
development, sweat, and elation.
Whether it's a run, a dance class, or a dip,
actual work discharges endorphins - your
body's regular pressure relievers.

5. Craftsmanship and Inventiveness:
Communicating Emotions
Envision your feelings as varieties ready
to be painted onto a material.
Craftsmanship and imagination become

your range, empowering you to communicate sentiments that words can't catch. Whether it's painting, composing, or making, these exercises offer a source for pressure, changing it into substantial manifestations of magnificence.

6. Social Help: The Force of Connection
Imagine yourself encompassed by a circle of help, where your pressure is met with sympathy and understanding. Social associations become your help, whether it's trusting in a companion, going to help gatherings, or looking for proficient direction. Sharing your encounters eases up the weight of pressure, making the excursion more tolerable.

7. Nature and Unwinding: Embracing the Outdoors
Imagine yourself drenched in the quietness of nature, away from the

requests of day to day existence. Nature turns into your safe-haven, offering comfort and point of view. Whether it's a comfortable walk around the recreation area, a climb in the forest, or basically sitting by the water, associating with nature revives your soul and lightens pressure.

As you dive into this section, perceive that pressure on the board isn't simply a procedure - it's an excursion toward recovering your profound prosperity. These strategies aren't simply instruments; they're the extension between the difficulties of today and the potential outcomes of tomorrow. By embracing pressure the board, you're not simply upgrading your ripeness process; you're making an ensemble of equilibrium, flexibility, and trust that resounds with the commitment of new life.

Exercise, Rest, and Hormonal Equilibrium: A Ternion for Ripeness Empowerment

In the ensemble of fruitfulness, three central participants - exercise, rest, and hormonal equilibrium - create an agreeable ternion that organizes the beat of regenerative wellbeing. This section is an investigation of their interconnected jobs, uncovering how each note adds to the piece of ripeness strengthening.

1. Exercise: The Movement of Hormones Envision practice as the choreographer, directing hormonal artists fitting together amazingly. Participating in standard actual work doesn't simply shape your physical make-up; it leads a

hormonal orchestra that upholds ovulation, directs insulin levels, and cultivates a decent feminine cycle. The dance of activity additionally sustains flow, conveying supplements to conceptive organs and guaranteeing their ideal capability.

2. Sleep: The Supportive Lullaby
Imagine rest as a mitigating cradlesong that supports your body, brain, and ripeness goals. During rest, your body fixes and revives, and your endocrine framework discharges chemicals fundamental for conceptive wellbeing. Sufficient rest upholds the equilibrium of key fruitfulness chemicals like luteinizing chemical (LH) and follicle-animating chemical (FSH), guaranteeing that your body's ensemble plays in amazing tune.

3. Hormonal Equilibrium: The Maestro's Baton

Imagine hormonal equilibrium as the maestro's cudgel, organizing the complex hormonal interaction fundamental for richness. Chemicals like estrogen, progesterone, and testosterone become the dominant focal point, directing ovulation, supporting pregnancies, and keeping up with contraceptive wellbeing. Exercise and rest become your partners in keeping up with this fragile equilibrium, guaranteeing that the hormonal group performs with accuracy.

4. Exercise, Rest, and Hormonal Synchronization: A Captivating Trio Picture the three components as interlocking pinion wheels that synchronize your body's complicated apparatus. Taking part in normal activity improves rest quality as well as supports hormonal equilibrium. Rest, thus, fills your energy for workout, while hormonal equilibrium cultivates more peaceful rest.

This charming threesome blossoms with a recurrent relationship, every component improving the others in an ensemble of ripeness enhancement.

5. Making Your Fruitfulness Ensemble: Commonsense Strategies
Envision this section as a writer's aide, offering down to earth procedures to blend the group of three. Take part in moderate activity that reverberates with your body, whether it's yoga, lively strolls, or strength preparing. Make a rest safe-haven by laying out a standard rest plan and rehearsing unwinding strategies. Focus on entire food varieties that feed hormonal wellbeing, and consider counseling a medical care proficient for customized direction.

As you dig into this part, recollect that activity, rest, and hormonal equilibrium are not confined notes; they're the cornerstones of a richness concerto that reverberates with imperativeness. By sustaining this set of three, you're not simply improving your possibilities of origination; you're creating a song of prosperity that reverberates through each fiber of your being. Welcome to the domain where exercise, rest, and hormonal equilibrium join to enable your fruitfulness process with elegance, strength, and the commitment of new life.

CONTENT 5. Holistic Approaches

All encompassing Methodologies: Sustaining Fruitfulness from Within

In the embroidered artwork of fruitfulness, all encompassing methodologies arise as the directing string that winds around together the physical, profound, and otherworldly components of your excursion. This part fills in as a dazzling survey of the comprehensive scene, where you'll find a mother lode of techniques that rise above the limits of regular reasoning. Plan to leave on an excursion that embraces your entire being, as you reveal the force of comprehensive methodologies in sustaining richness from the inside.

1. Mind-Body Association: The Inward Sanctuary
Envision your psyche and body as a fragile biological system, where concordance is the way to fruitfulness. All encompassing methodologies perceive this significant association, offering strategies like reflection, perception, and profound breathing to overcome any issues between your viewpoints and your actual prosperity. By developing internal harmony, you're making a ripe ground for your fantasies of life as a parent to flourish.

2. Nourishing Concordance: Taking care of Fertility
Imagine your body as a material, hanging tight for the brushstrokes of supplement

rich food sources to portray imperativeness. Comprehensive sustenance extends past calories and macros, digging into the helpful capability of entire food varieties, spices, and enhancements that sustain fruitfulness at its center. This approach recognizes the significant effect of sustenance on chemicals, conceptive organs, and generally speaking health.

3. Natural Partners: Nature's Remedies
Picture nature as your partner, offering a different cluster of spices that can uphold your richness process. All encompassing methodologies tap into the mending capability of botanicals like chasteberry, maca, and red raspberry leaf, each conveying interesting properties that reverberate with regenerative health. These spices become your accomplices, directing you toward hormonal equilibrium and imperativeness.

4. Needle therapy and Conventional Medication: Energy Flow
Envision pathways of energy flowing through your body, affected by antiquated rehearses that look to reestablish harmony. Comprehensive methodologies consolidate needle therapy, Customary Chinese Medication, and Ayurveda, all of which perceive the significance of energy stream for richness. Through these modalities, you tap into centuries old insight that adjusts your body's energies to your desires.

5. Close to home Prosperity: Divulging Internal Strength
Imagine your feelings as varieties ready to be recognized, communicated, and changed. Comprehensive methodologies dive into the domain of profound prosperity, offering devices like care, journaling, and helpful practices to

explore the close to home intricacies of the ripeness venture. By recognizing your sentiments and sustaining your soul, you're supporting richness from the inside.

6. Bodywork and Development: Active Healing
Picture your body as a vessel, receptive to the recuperating bit of all encompassing treatments. From back rub and reflexology to chiropractic care and craniosacral treatment, these methodologies tap into the intrinsic insight of your body, delivering strain and supporting prosperity. Through development rehearsals like yoga and qigong, you orchestrate the energy stream and encourage an open climate for origination.

7. Proficient Direction: Master Compass

Imagine comprehensive specialists as guides on your excursion, offering aptitude that spans ordinary medication with elective methodologies. These experts tailor their suggestions to your exceptional necessities, guaranteeing that your all encompassing way is lined up with your clinical history, objectives, and values.

As you ponder this part, recall that comprehensive methodologies are not simply individual strategies; they're interconnected features of a multi-layered way to deal with richness. By embracing the all encompassing domain, you're venturing into an existence where each part of your being is regarded, where your process isn't only about origination, yet about change, strengthening, and the acknowledgment of your most profound desires. Welcome to the domain of all encompassing methodologies, where your process turns into an embroidery of prosperity that resounds with the commitment of life itself.

Mind-Body Association: Sustaining Richness Through Reflection and Visualization

Envision a domain where your considerations have the ability to shape your world, where your psyche turns into a material whereupon your fruitfulness process unfurls. This section is a challenge to investigate the significant scene of the brain body association, where reflection and representation arise as your devices to orchestrate considerations and physiology, encouraging a climate of prosperity and fruitfulness.

1. Meditation: An Excursion Inward
Imagine yourself in a quiet safe-haven,
liberated from the jabber of day to day
existence. Reflection turns into your
pathway to this inward desert spring,
directing you toward a condition of care
and presence. As you calm your psyche,
you tap into the helpful force of
unwinding, lessening pressure and
permitting your body to flourish.

2. Care Reflection: Securing in the
Present
Envision your considerations as passing
mists, while your mindfulness remains
secured right now. Care contemplation
turns into your work, preparing you to
notice considerations without judgment.
By embracing the present time and place,
you discharge the hold of stresses over
the past and nerves about the future,

making mental space for fruitfulness'
capability to prosper.

3. Directed Symbolism: Painting Your Fruitfulness Dreams

Imagine yourself as the craftsman of your ripeness process, using the brush of directed symbolism. This strategy takes you on an excursion through striking mental scenes, moving you to peaceful spots where your cravings for being a parent can show. As you draw in your faculties in this psychological embroidered artwork, your body answers by blending with your envisioned expectations.

4. Visualization: Making Ripe Realities

Imaginc the future as a material yet to be painted, where your imagination holds the brush of perception. With centered expectation, you can direct your contemplations to picture the origination, pregnancy, and birth you want. Perception takes advantage of the psyche's ability to impact the body, adjusting chemicals and physiological reactions to your fantasies.

5. Close to home Reverberation: Treating Internal Soil
Envision feelings as rich soil, ready to be fed by the waters of good representation. By imbuing your representations with feelings of happiness, trust, and appreciation, you extend the association among the brain and body. This close to home reverberation conveys messages that echo through your framework, developing a climate helpful for origination.

6. Brain connections: Revamping the Script
Imagine your mind as a nursery, where your considerations plant seeds that

develop into brain processes. Reflection and perception become your instruments for developing pathways that help richness. By revamping negative idea designs into positive assertions, you engage your psyche to team up with your body's desires.

7. Practice and Tolerance: Supporting the Brain Body Seedling
Picture your psyche body association as a seedling that requires sustaining and persistence. Reliable act of reflection and representation cultivates development, with benefits stretching out past fruitfulness. Diminished pressure, worked on close to home prosperity, and upgraded mind-body synchronization become the blooms of your devotion.

As you dive into this section, recollect that reflection and representation are not simply strategies; they're passages to the further elements of your fruitfulness process. By supporting this psyche body association, you're keeping an eye on the foundations of your fantasies, implanting your way with aim, and cultivating a full climate where origination can flourish. Welcome to the domain where your contemplations become your partners, forming a prolific reality that orchestrates with your deepest longings.

Conventional Practices and Elective Treatments: Uncovering Richness' Secret Pathways

In the complicated mosaic of ripeness, customary practices and elective treatments arise as the secret pathways that lead you toward an embroidery of prosperity. This section fills in as a charming survey, welcoming you to investigate the rich embroidery of approaches that rise above regular medication. Here, you'll reveal the insight of old customs and imaginative treatments that offer new points of view on your richness process.

1. Antiquated Insight: Reverberations of Time
Envision your process crossing with the reverberations of previous eras, as customary practices are uncovered as ageless fortunes. From Conventional Chinese Medication's needle therapy to Ayurveda's home grown cures, these well established frameworks perceive the significance of equilibrium in sustaining fruitfulness. By regarding their insight, you're taking advantage of the aggregate encounters of the individuals who preceded.

2\. Home grown Partners: Nature's Resonance

Imagine nature as an ensemble of mending, with spices as its sweet notes. Elective treatments tackle the force of botanicals like night primrose oil, dong quai, and vitex to help hormonal harmony, regenerative organ wellbeing, and feminine cycle consistency. Every spice turns into an instrument in the ensemble of ripeness, fitting your excursion.

3\. Energy Stream: Old Pathways

Envision your body as an organization of pathways where energy streams, ready to be adjusted. Customary practices like needle therapy and Reiki dive into the domain of energy, unblocking stale streams and cultivating a fair climate for origination. These treatments offer a comprehensive viewpoint, perceiving the interconnectedness of your body, brain, and soul.

4. Mind-Body Congruity: Inward Sanctuary

Imagine the sanctum of your psyche as a fruitful ground, prepared to embrace old practices that fit your contemplations with your body's rhythms. Reflection, yoga, and perception become your instruments, encouraging unwinding, decreasing pressure, and making a psychological space that resounds with ripeness' true capacity.

5. Development and Articulation: Body's Language

Picture your body's developments as a language, recounting an account of recuperating and change. Dance treatment, substantial encountering, and expressive expressions welcome you to investigate the stories held inside your body, offering a way to deliver feelings, develop mindfulness, and improve profound prosperity.

6. Proficient Direction: The Scaffold to Balance

Imagine elective specialists as scaffolds among traditional and comprehensive methodologies, offering an abundance of mastery that lines up with your novel necessities. Whether it's looking for a naturopath, cultivator, or energy healer, their direction turns into your compass in exploring these unfamiliar pathways.

7. Individual Strengthening: Another Frontier

Consider the capability of mixing customary practices and elective treatments with regular medication. This combination welcomes you to recover office over your ripeness process, embracing a complete methodology that praises both science and comprehensive insight.

As you mull over this section, recall that customary practices and elective treatments are not dissimilar ways; they're features of a multi-layered way to deal with ripeness. By embracing these secret pathways, you're opening yourself to a domain where potential outcomes are limitless, where old information meets current comprehension. Welcome to the universe of customary practices and elective treatments - a domain where the combination of shrewdness and innovation leads you toward an excursion that resounds with change, strengthening, and the commitment of new life.

CONTENT.6.Medical Insights

Clinical Bits of knowledge: Enlightening Ripeness' Way with Science

Step into the domain where current science converges with the desires of life as a parent - the section of Clinical Experiences. Here, the cover of vulnerability is lifted as we explore through the complexities of conceptual wellbeing, disclosing the clinical points of view that shed light on your fruitfulness process. Get ready to set out on an excursion where information turns into your compass, directing you through the intricacies of origination with lucidity, strengthening, and trust.

1. The Contraceptive Ensemble: Chemicals and Ovulation
Envision your body as an ensemble symphony, with chemicals as the directors that arrange ovulation's sensitive dance. Clinical experiences dig into the hormonal interchange that arranges the period - from follicle-animating chemical (FSH) directing follicle development to luteinizing chemical (LH) setting off ovulation. Understanding this orchestra engages you to distinguish ideal richness windows.

2. Ripeness Diagnostics: Disclosing Insights
Picture fruitfulness diagnostics as the amplifying glass that uncovers the unpredictable activities of your

conceptual framework. Clinical innovation offers instruments like ultrasound, blood tests, and imaging, permitting you to follow follicular turn of events, evaluate egg quality, and screen hormonal equilibrium. These experiences become your friends, directing choices and upgrading your way.

3. Helped Conceptive Advances (Craftsmanship): Exploring Options Imagine Workmanship as a domain where science meets trust, offering a range of answers for different challenges. From intrauterine insemination (IUI) to in vitro treatment (IVF), these procedures give potential chances to conquer boundaries to origination. Clinical experiences guide you in understanding the methodology, achievement rates, and contemplations for every choice.

4. Male Fruitfulness: The Other Portion of the Equation

Envision ripeness as a riddle with two parts, where male elements are similarly critical. Clinical experiences into male ripeness investigate sperm quality, amount, and morphology. By figuring out the effect of way of life, hereditary qualities, and wellbeing on sperm, you embrace an exhaustive methodology that thinks about the two accomplices.

5. Hormonal Uneven characters: Opening Causes and Solutions

Imagine hormonal uneven characters as riddles ready to be settled. Clinical bits of knowledge uncover conditions like polycystic ovary condition (PCOS), endometriosis, and thyroid problems that can influence fruitfulness. Equipped with information, you team up with clinical experts to investigate custom-made arrangements that address the fundamental causes.

6. Previously established inclination Care: Sustaining Ripeness' Soil
Picture predisposition care as the foundation for a solid pregnancy. Clinical bits of knowledge guide you through way of life changes, wholesome contemplations, and supplementation to improve your body for origination. By setting up your body, you establish a climate where the seeds of new life can prosper.

7. Profound Prosperity: Incorporating Science and Mind
Envision clinical bits of knowledge as a scaffold that interfaces your close to home prosperity with logical comprehension. Clinical experts recognize the close to home parts of the fruitfulness venture, offering backing and

direction to address pressure, tension, and emotional wellness. This mix engages you to explore the physiological, yet additionally the close to home scene of richness.

As you retain the data in this section, recall that clinical experiences are not simply information; they're guides that enlighten your way toward being a parent. By coordinating science with your desires, you're embracing an excursion of informed decisions, cooperation with clinical experts, and strengthening. Welcome to the domain where clinical bits of knowledge become your compass, driving you toward a richness venture that reverberates with figuring out, certainty, and the commitment of new life.

Clinical Intercessions and Helped Contraceptive Advancements: Spearheading Pathways to Parenthood

In the scene of fruitfulness, science reveals its most complex embroidered works of art through the sections of Clinical Mediations and Helped Conceptive Advancements (Craftsmanship). This section fills in as an enthralling survey, offering you a directed visit through the domain where clinical development meets the desires of being a parent. Here, you'll investigate the roads that enable you to explore richness challenges earnestly, trust, and logical understanding.

1. Richness Medicines: Disclosing Possibilities

Envision fruitful medicines as a range of conceivable outcomes, each shade addressing a remarkable way to deal with understanding your fantasy of life as a parent. Clinical mediations range from ovulation enlistment to medical procedure, tending to conditions that influence fruitfulness. With clinical bits of knowledge as your compass, you team up with medical care experts to plan a custom-made approach that suits your necessities.

2. Intrauterine Insemination (IUI): Arranging Conception
Picture IUI as an orchestra director, adjusting sperm and egg to fit in the dance of origination. This helped regenerative innovation include putting extraordinarily pre-arranged sperm straightforwardly into the uterus, improving the possibilities of treatment. Clinical experiences guide you through the interaction, achievement rates, and

contemplations, engaging you with
information.

3. In Vitro Treatment (IVF): An
Excursion of Hope
Imagine IVF as an excursion of trust,
where science and assurance meet to
sustain life. This progressive
Workmanship includes treating eggs with
sperm outside the body and moving
incipient organisms into the uterus.
Clinical experiences enlighten the means,
from ovarian feeling and egg recovery to
incipient organism move, demystifying
the cycle and enabling you.

4. Intracytoplasmic Sperm Infusion
(ICSI): Accuracy in Creation
Envision ICSI as a sensitive expert,
putting a solitary sperm into an egg with
fastidious accuracy. This method,
frequently utilized related to IVF, beats
male barrenness challenges. Clinical bits

of knowledge give a window into ICSI's groundbreaking potential, featuring its part in conquering obstructions to origination.

5. Contributor Origination: Embracing New Paths

Picture giver origination as an extension to being a parent, offering desire to people and couples confronting explicit difficulties. Whether utilizing giver sperm, eggs, or incipient organisms, clinical bits of knowledge guide you through the contemplations, legalities, and profound subtleties of this way, engaging you to pursue informed choices.

6. Hereditary Screening: Spearheading Precision

Imagine hereditary screening as a compass that guides you toward a solid pregnancy. Preimplantation hereditary testing (PGT) evaluates undeveloped organisms for hereditary problems before implantation, upgrading the possibilities of an effective pregnancy. Clinical bits of knowledge enlighten this state of the art innovation, giving a brief look into its true capacity and contemplations.

7. Close to home Strength: Incorporating Science and Hope
Envision clinical mediations and Workmanship as scaffolds among science and the human soul. This part recognizes the profound excursion, offering bits of knowledge into guiding, supporting gatherings, and methodologies to explore the ups and downs. By embracing profound flexibility, you're setting out on a logical undertaking, yet in addition an extraordinary way of strengthening and development.

As you ponder this part, recall that clinical mediations and Craftsmanship are not simply systems; they're excursions of strengthening, science, and trust. By coordinating these pathways with your yearnings, you're leaving on a complex experience that reverberates sincerely, educated decisions, and the commitment of new life. Welcome to the domain where clinical intercessions and helped conceptual innovations become your partners, driving you toward a ripeness venture that blends science and the human soul.

Master Exhortation: Exploring the Way to Clinical Assistance with Confidence

Envision a compass in your grasp, directing you toward an objective of clearness and trust. This part, Master

Exhortation, fills in as your compass, guiding you toward clinical assistance with steadfast certainty. Here, you'll reveal the bits of knowledge that engage you to perceive when to look for clinical help, how to explore the medical services scene, and how to team up successfully with experts on your richness process.

1. Confiding in Your Instinct: Signs to Look for Help
Picture your instinct as a murmur, delicately encouraging you to perceive when help is required. Master exhortation urges you to pay attention to your body's prompts - unpredictable cycles, industrious agony, or close to home misery - and view them as signs to look for clinical direction. By recognizing these signs, you venture out toward strengthening.

2. Essential Consideration Doctors: Your Underlying Guides

Envision your essential consideration doctor as your most memorable aide on this excursion. Master exhortation urges you to share your interests straightforwardly, as they can start fundamental tests and assessments. If necessary, they'll allude you to subject matter experts, guaranteeing that your clinical excursion is secured in joint effort and extensive consideration.

3. Ripeness Subject matter experts: Exploring the Landscape

Picture richness experts as talented guides through the landscape of contraceptive wellbeing. Master exhortation guides you in choosing a richness center, investigating factors like achicvement rates, patient tributes, and customized approaches. These experts become accomplices who tailor

medicines to your necessities, strolling
alongside you on the way to life as a
parent.

4. Appraisals and Diagnostics: Bits of
knowledge Unveiled
Imagine clinical appraisals as keys that
open bits of knowledge into your ripeness
puzzle. Master exhortation urges you to
be proactive in going through tests that
assess hormonal equilibrium, egg quality,
sperm wellbeing, and contraceptive
organ usefulness. Furnished with this
data, you're prepared to pursue informed
choices.

5. Customized Plans: Coordinated effort
in Care
Envision clinical experts as planners,
planning customized plans that line up
with your goals. Master exhortation
highlights the significance of dynamic
cooperation, talking about treatment

choices, achievement rates, dangers, and possible results. By participating in straightforward discussions, you're effectively forming your ripeness process.

6. Profound Prosperity: Respecting Your Journey

Picture your close to home prosperity as a foundation of your richness. Master guidance stresses the benefit of looking for everyday encouragement, whether through directing, treatment, or care groups. By recognizing your feelings and supporting your psychological wellness, you're cultivating strength that upgrades your clinical excursion.

7. Second Suppositions: Embracing Informed Choices

Envision second sentiments as designated spots that engage you to pursue informed decisions. Master guidance empowers looking for extra viewpoints if necessary, guaranteeing that you're positive about the proposals you get. By embracing various bits of knowledge, you're enabled to pursue choices that resound with your qualities and objectives.

As you ponder this part, recall that looking for clinical assistance isn't simply a stage; it's a demonstration of self-strengthening. By embracing master counsel, you're leaving on an excursion where coordinated effort, information, and trust join together. This excursion, moored in your assurance and the direction of experts, leads you toward a fruitful way that resounds with certainty, understanding, and the commitment of new life.

CONTENT 7. Fertility Tracking and Ovulation

Fruitfulness Following and Ovulation: Exploring the Enormous Dance of Conception

In the universe of ripeness, following your body's rhythms and understanding the complexities of ovulation resemble outlining the heavenly dance of stars. This section, Ripeness Following and Ovulation, welcomes you to investigate the science and specialty of fruitfulness mindfulness, offering experiences that enable you to synchronize your endeavors with the universe's amazing plan. Plan to set out on an excursion of self-disclosure, where you'll uncover the secret examples that guide your way toward origination.

1. Monthly cycle: The Rhythms of Creation
Envision your feminine cycle as a grandiose orchestra, each stage a note that leads you nearer to the crescendo of ovulation. Fruitfulness following uncovers this mood, engaging you to perceive the follicular stage's development and the luteal stage's hormonal organization. By understanding your cycle's rhythmic movement, you're receptive to your body's mysterious language.

2. Basal Internal heat level (BBT): Graphing the Shifts

Picture your basal internal heat level as a thermometer of richness, its variances uncovering the orchestra of hormonal movements. Fruitfulness following includes taking your temperature every morning to distinguish the temperature climb that signals ovulation. This method offers a window into your cycle's subtleties, enabling you to time closeness with accuracy.

3. Cervical Bodily fluid: Nature's Indicator

Imagine cervical bodily fluid as nature's compass, directing you toward the fruitful territory of ovulation. Ripeness following urges you to notice the progressions in bodily fluid consistency and variety, from dry to clear and stretchy. This unmistakable marker turns into your aide, featuring your body's preparation for origination.

4. Ovulation Indicator Packs (OPKs): Holding onto the Moment
Envision OPKs as enormous couriers, flagging the perfect second for origination. These packs recognize the flood of luteinizing chemicals (LH) that go before ovulation. Fruitfulness following OPKs turns into your apparatus for pinpointing the window of richness, guaranteeing that you're prepared to embrace the grandiose dance of creation.

5. Fruitfulness Applications and Screens: Innovation's Harmony
Picture ripeness applications and screens as present day groups of stars, directing your excursion with innovation's touch. These apparatuses group information, anticipating prolific days and ovulation with calculations. Fruitfulness following turns into a computerized orchestra, where you input your perceptions and get

experiences that line up with your inestimable goals.

6. Cervical Position: Measuring Richness' Terrain

Envision your cervix as a compass that movements with your cycle's rhythms. Ripeness following includes noticing changes in the cervix's situation, surface, and receptiveness. By understanding these signs, you become sensitive to the astronomical timing of richness, exploring toward the gravitational draw of origination.

7. Profound Association: Fruitfulness' Inestimable Bond

Envision your profound association with your body as the inestimable bond that rises above information. Fruitfulness following turns into an excursion of mindfulness, encouraging closeness with your body's rhythms. By embracing this association, you're not simply noticing the infinite dance; you're a member in its creation.

As you investigate this part, recall that richness following and understanding ovulation are not simply methods; they're entryways to a more profound association with your body and the universe. By orchestrating your endeavors with the universe, you're venturing into a domain where science and instinct join together, directing you toward an excursion that reverberates with accuracy, arrangement, and the commitment of new life. Welcome to the vast dance of richness following and ovulation - an excursion where you become a divine guide of creation.

Dominating Your Feminine cycle: Ovulation Expectation Unveiled

In the ensemble of fruitfulness, understanding your period resembles translating the melodic examples that lead to the crescendo of ovulation. This part, "Dominating Your Feminine cycle: Ovulation Expectation," fills in as your aide through the mind boggling notes and harmonies that form your body's beat. Here, you'll uncover the insider facts of ovulation expectation, empowering you to adjust your endeavors to the basic dance of creation.

1. The Cycle's Ensemble: A Preface to Ovulation

Envision your feminine cycle as a melodic score, each stage adding to the amicable ensemble of fruitfulness. Ovulation forecast starts with perceiving your cycle's rhythmic movement - from period to the follicular stage's crescendo and the luteal stage's goal. By adjusting yourself to these stages, you're prepared to anticipate the climactic snapshot of ovulation.

2. Basal Internal heat level (BBT): The Temperature Prelude
Picture your basal internal heat level as the initial note of ovulation expectation. BBT following includes estimating your temperature after waking every day, uncovering unobtrusive movements that show hormonal changes. As your cycle advances, a temperature climb flags ovulation's methodology. This technique enables you to anticipate your prolific window with accuracy.

3. Ovulation Indicator Packs (OPKs): The Consonant Surge
Envision OPKs as the guide's stick, directing you toward the pinnacle of

fruitfulness. These packs recognize the flood of luteinizing chemicals (LH) that goes before ovulation, anticipating the second when your body is prepared for origination. By utilizing OPKs, you're embracing a strategy that blends your endeavors with your body's intrinsic musicality.

4. Cervical Bodily fluid: The Ripe Crescendo

Picture cervical bodily fluid as the crescendo of richness, showing the ideal circumstances for origination. Ovulation forecast includes noticing changes in bodily fluid surface and consistency - from dry to clear and stretchy. This perceptible pointer guides you toward your prolific window, permitting you to expect the inestimable dance of ovulation.

5. Feminine Applications and Screens: Innovation's Serenade

Imagine feminine applications and screens as the computerized notices that reverberate with innovation's touch. These devices group your cycle information, foreseeing fruitful days and ovulation with algorithmic accuracy. Ovulation forecast turns into an amicable combination of science and present day comfort, as you input information and get experiences lined up with your body's song.

6. Cervical Position: The Physical Prelude

Picture your cervix as the instrument that resounds with your cycle's rhythms. Ovulation expectation includes following changes in the cervix's situation, surface, and receptiveness. As you ace this strategy, you're receptive to the physical prompts that foretell the grandiose ensemble of ovulation.

7. Individual Strengthening: The Guide of Conception

Envision yourself as the guide of your fruitfulness process, flawlessly coordinating ovulation forecast methods. By dominating your monthly cycle, you're assuming control over your excursion, coordinating your endeavors toward the agreeable objective of origination. This dominance turns into a demonstration of your assurance and association with the basic rhythms of life.

As you dig into this part, recall that ovulation forecast isn't simply an expertise; it's a work of art that spans science and instinct. By dominating your feminine cycle, you're venturing into a domain where you orchestrate your desires with your body's song. Welcome to the universe of ovulation forecast - an excursion of revelation, arrangement, and the commitment of fresh starts.

Graphing Basal Internal heat level and Cervical Bodily fluid: Translating Nature's Richness Symphony

Envision your body as a stupendous ensemble, where the subtlest notes of basal internal heat level (BBT) and cervical bodily fluid make an orchestra that guides you through the mind boggling dance of richness. This section plunges profoundly into the specialty of graphing BBT and noticing cervical bodily fluid, divulging the secret rhythms that hold the way to foreseeing ovulation with accuracy. Get ready to submerge yourself in the agreeable language of your body, as you figure out how to decipher nature's richness ensemble.

1. Basal Internal heat level (BBT): The Temperature Canvas
Imagine BBT as the material whereupon your richness process unfurls. Graphing BBT includes taking your temperature after waking every morning, catching the unobtrusive movements that reflect hormonal changes all through your feminine cycle. As you record these temperatures, an example arises - a delicate ascent showing ovulation's methodology. This creative practice enables you to anticipate your prolific window and hold onto the incredible luck for origination.

2. Cervical Bodily fluid: Nature's Liquid Poetry
Picture cervical bodily fluid as nature's liquid verse, offering experiences into

your body's fruitfulness scene. Outlining cervical bodily fluid includes noticing its surface, variety, and consistency all through your cycle. From dry days to damp, tacky, lastly to clear and stretchy, these varieties reflect your hormonal changes. This melodious practice guides you toward your ripe days, making a guide to ovulation.

3. The Diagramming System: Following the Patterns

Envision your ripeness graph as a melodic score, with every day's BBT and cervical bodily fluid perceptions shaping the notes that create your body's song. As you outline these perceptions on diagram paper or with computerized devices, you reveal designs one of a kind to your cycle. Tops in BBT and the advances in cervical bodily fluid become the crescendos that envoys ovulation's appearance.

4. Design Acknowledgment: Coordinating Ovulation

Picture yourself as the director of your fruitfulness orchestra, receptive to the subtleties of example acknowledgment. By dissecting your BBT and cervical bodily fluid diagram, you'll distinguish the shift that signals ovulation. The agreement between raised BBT, rich quality cervical bodily fluid, and different signs turns into your guidepost, guiding you to your ideal origination window.

5. Strengthening Through Information: Tuning In

Envision strengthening as the reverberation that comes from figuring out your body's exceptional rhythms. Graphing BBT and cervical bodily fluid changes you into a functioning member in your richness process. This close information permits you to expect your ripe days, adjusting your endeavors to the inestimable dance of origination.

6. Accomplice Contribution: A Two part harmony of Support

Picture your accomplice as a colleague in this orchestra of fruitfulness. Imparting your diagram and bits of knowledge to them encourages a feeling of shared liability and backing. Together, you're arranging the excursion toward life as a parent, orchestrating your endeavors and goals.

7. Profound Association: The Heartbeat of Fertility

Imagine your close to home association with diagramming as the heartbeat that synchronizes with your body's mood. This training goes past information; it cultivates closeness with your body's normal cycles. By embracing this association, you're supporting your ripeness process as well as your relationship with yourself.

As you dive into the specialty of graphing BBT and cervical bodily fluid, recollect that you're setting out on an excursion of revelation and strengthening. This excursion reverberates with the agreement among science and instinct, where your body turns into your aide, and nature's orchestra turns into your motivation. Welcome to the existence where outlining BBT and noticing cervical bodily fluid permit you to reveal the secret examples that lead you toward a fruitful way lined up with the rhythms of creation.

CONTENT . 8. Creating a Fertility-Friendly Environment

Establishing a Climate that welcomes richnesses: Developing the Nursery of Conception

Envision your body as a nursery, anticipating the supporting touch that changes it into a prolific safe-haven. This part, "Establishing a Ripeness Accommodating Climate," welcomes you to step into the job of a grounds-keeper, watching out for the dirt of your body and environmental elements to establish a climate helpful for origination. Here, you'll investigate the all encompassing viewpoints that orchestrate to cultivate fruitfulness, from way of life changes in accordance with home adjustments. Get ready to develop a nursery of prosperity, where the seeds of new life can thrive.

1. Nutrition: Planting Seeds of Nourishment
Picture nourishment as the supplements that enhance your body's dirt. By consolidating a fair eating routine plentiful in nutrients, minerals, cell reinforcements, and omega-3 unsaturated fats, you're sustaining a climate where chemicals flourish and conceptual organs capability ideally. This culinary consideration engages you to develop a ripe starting point for origination.

2. Hydration: Extinguishing the Hunger for Fertility
Envision hydration as the water that supports the foundations of your

ripeness. Remaining sufficiently hydrated upholds cervical bodily fluid creation, supporting sperm's excursion toward the egg. By tasting water over the course of the day, you're watching out for the nursery of your body, guaranteeing it stays a fruitful safe house for the capability of new life.

3. Overseeing Pressure: Removing Tension

Picture pressure as the weeds that take steps to choke out your ripe garden. Establishing a fruitfulness accommodating climate includes rehearsing pressure decrease strategies like contemplation, profound breathing, and yoga. By getting rid of stressors, you're making space for unwinding, hormonal equilibrium, and an environment where origination can flourish.

4. Sleep: Keeping an eye on the Dirt of Rest

Envision rest as the supportive rest that sustains the dirt of your body. Focusing on quality rest upholds hormonal balance and in general prosperity. By developing solid rest propensities, you're encouraging a climate where your body's rhythms adjust agreeably, preparing for fruitfulness to thrive.

5. Poison Decrease: Clearing the Path

Envision poisons as the obstructions that ruin your ripeness process. Establishing a ripeness accommodating climate includes lessening openness to ecological poisons, like synthetics in private consideration items and pesticides in food. By making the way of these obstructions, you're making an unadulterated space for origination to happen.

6. Actual work: Developing Movement Picture actual work as the movement that strengthens your rich garden. Taking part in normal activity upholds blood flow, hormonal equilibrium, and profound prosperity. By developing development in your everyday daily practice, you're improving the rich climate inside your body, empowering the seeds of origination to thrive.

7. Home Climate: Upgrading Harmony Envision your home climate as the safe-haven that supports your ripeness. Making a fruitfulness accommodating space includes limiting openness to endocrine-disturbing synthetics, advancing great indoor air quality, and embracing unwinding through relieving style. By organizing an amicable home, you're encouraging a climate where richness is normally upheld.

8. Closeness and Association: Treating the Heart

Picture closeness as the demonstration that prepares the body as well as the heart. Establishing a ripeness accommodating climate includes supporting close to home associations with your accomplice. By cultivating a cherishing, steady relationship, you're improving the dirt of your excursion, making a space where both love and life can flourish.

As you dive into the craft of establishing a ripeness accommodating climate, recall that you're leaving on an excursion of all encompassing prosperity. By sustaining your body, psyche, and environmental factors, you're developing a space where the seeds of origination are greeted wholeheartedly. This excursion resounds with the magnificence of equilibrium, the force of expectation, and the commitment of new life. Welcome to the existence where you become the landscaper of your richness, keeping an eye on the nursery of potential with care, commitment, and the significant association among nature and support.

Poison Free Living: Embracing Nature's Concordance in a Cutting edge World

Envision your life as a fragile biological system, where the decisions echo through your current circumstance and prosperity. This section, "Poison Free Living," coaxes you to step into the job of a steward for both your body and the planet. Here, you'll leave on an excursion that interlaces wellbeing and maintainability, divulging the force of limiting natural poisons. Get ready to drench yourself in the specialty of poison free residing, where nature's congruity flourishes inside the cutting edge world.

1. Natural Effect: A Wave Effect
Picture your decisions as stones cast into the waters of your life, making swells that reach out a long way past your nearby environmental elements. Poison free living recognizes the interconnectedness between private prosperity and the strength of the planet. By limiting openness to poisons, you're adding to a cleaner environment, helping yourself as well as people in the future.

2. Endocrine Disruptors: Exposing the Culprits
Envision endocrine disruptors as concealed strings that upset the sensitive woven artwork of your body's hormonal equilibrium. Poison free living includes recognizing and keeping away from these troublesome mixtures, generally tracked

down in plastics, pesticides, and certain beauty care products. By exposing these offenders, you're supporting a rich climate inside your body and safeguarding the world's sensitive biological systems.

3. Regular Other options: Regarding Earth's Bounty
Picture normal choices as gifts from the earth, giving sustenance to both body and planet. Poison free living empowers the utilization of regular cleaning items, natural food sources, and eco-accommodating individual consideration things. By embracing these other options, you're deciding to blend with nature's rhythms, lessening your environmental impression.

4. Home Climate: A Safe-haven of Purity
Picture your home as a safe-haven where poison free residing prospers. Limiting

natural poisons includes decontaminating indoor air quality, disposing of manufactured scents, and picking eco-accommodating materials. By developing a space that praises your wellbeing and the planet, you're making a shelter where prosperity flourishes.

5. Careful Utilization: Stepping Lightly Envision careful utilization as a way that follows the effect of your decisions from creation to removal. Poison free living includes picking items with insignificant bundling, supporting maintainable practices, and reusing things whenever the situation allows. By proceeding with caution on the earth, you're adding to an existence where poisons have less of an open door to invade.

6. Excellence and Individual Consideration: Embracing Regular Elegance

Picture excellence and individual consideration items as expansions of your poison free living excursion. Settle on beauty care products, skincare, and cleanliness things that focus on regular, natural fixings. By embracing items that honor your body's prosperity, you're upgrading your wellbeing while at the same time encouraging a veneration for the climate.

7. Local area and Backing: A Brought together Voice

Envision poison free living as a development that accumulates strength through aggregate activity. Draw in with your local area to bring issues to light about the effect of poisons and promoters for cleaner rehearsals. By joining your voice with others, you're intensifying the need for a better world, where poison free residing turns into a common responsibility.

8. Empowerment: Developing Change
Envision yourself as an influencer inside
the woven artwork of poison free living.
By settling on informed decisions,
instructing others, and supporting
maintainable drives, you're developing a
culture where wellbeing and ecological
prosperity interweave. Your process
turns into a demonstration of the force of
individual activity in molding a more
splendid, cleaner future.

As you leave on the path of poison free
living, recall that you're not simply
settling on decisions for yourself; you're
impacting your general surroundings. By
embracing this excursion, you're fitting
with the rhythms of nature, defending
your prosperity, and leaving a tradition
of ecological stewardship. Welcome to
the domain where poison free residing
turns into an orchestra of wellbeing,

supportability, and the significant association between individual decisions and worldwide effect.

Home and Way of life Changes for Regenerative Wellbeing: Planning Your Prolific Haven

Envision your home as a material, hanging tight for the brushstrokes of goal that change it into a safe-haven of contraceptive wellbeing. This section, "Home and Way of life Changes for Regenerative Wellbeing," welcomes you to step into the job of a craftsman, organizing your environmental elements and day to day rhythms to fit with your fruitfulness process. Here, you'll investigate the manners by which your current circumstance and way of life can be changed in accordance with supporting conceptual prosperity. Get ready to set out on an excursion of comprehensive change, where your home and propensities become the establishment for richness' capability to thrive.

1. Comprehensive Supporting: An Outline for Wellness
Picture your home and way of life as the diagram whereupon your conceptive wellbeing is fabricated. This comprehensive methodology recognizes that wellbeing isn't exclusively about actual wellbeing; it reaches out to profound, mental, and otherworldly prosperity. By organizing your current circumstance and propensities, you're making an amicable space where all features of your being are sustained.

2. Green Living: Embracing Nature's Harmony

Envision green residing as a hug of nature's rhythms inside your home. Regenerative well being includes decreasing openness to harmful family items and embracing regular other options. From cleaning supplies to individual considerations, deciding on eco-accommodating decisions upholds your body's wellbeing while at the same time respecting the world's sensitive environments.

3. Careful Plan: Developing Tranquility Picture your home as a material for careful planning, cultivating a climate of quietness. Regenerative well being includes making spaces that advance unwinding and diminish pressure. Delicate varieties, normal surfaces, and quiet designs offer comfort to your faculties, permitting your psyche and body to loosen up and thrive.

4. Rest Safe-haven: Focusing on Rest
Envision your room as a rest safe-haven, a casing of solace that sustains your conceptive health. Focusing on serene rest includes establishing an ideal rest climate - from happy with bedding to limiting electronic gadgets before sleep time. By supporting your rest, you're cultivating hormonal equilibrium and revival.

5. Nourishment and Wellbeing: A Culinary Symphony
Picture sustenance as a culinary orchestra that upholds regenerative wellbeing. Careful eating includes devouring various supplement rich food sources that feed your body. Integrating cancer prevention agents, omega-3 unsaturated fats, and fruitfulness helping supplements energizes hormonal equilibrium and establishes an inner climate prepared for origination.

6. Development and Exercise: Stimulating Vitality

Picture development as the brushstroke that paints imperativeness across your material of regenerative health. Taking part in standard actual work upholds course, chemical guidelines, and close to home prosperity. From yoga to move, finding exercises that impact you improves your body's normal equilibrium.

7. Close to home Strength: The Heartbeat of Wellness

Envision profound strength as the heartbeat that reverberations inside your home and life. Conceptive wellbeing includes developing practices that help mental and profound wellbeing, like contemplation, care, and journaling. By embracing profound prosperity, you're making an inside scene that encourages fruitfulness and equilibrium.

8. Accomplice Association: Encouraging Unity
Picture your accomplice as a co-maker in the material of regenerative health. Sustaining your relationship includes open correspondence, shared exercises, and daily encouragement. By encouraging areas of strength for a, you're developing a climate of affection, understanding, and shared yearnings for a rich future.

As you dig into the domain of home and way of life changes for regenerative health, recollect that you're a craftsman molding your own prolific scene. By organizing your current circumstance and propensities, you're supporting an all encompassing sanctuary where your body, brain, and soul prosper. This excursion is a demonstration of the force of expectation, where your decisions blend with nature's rhythms and make the ideal scenery for the wonder of new life. Welcome to the existence where your home turns into a material of health, and your way of life turns into the brush that paints a lively way to regenerative prosperity.

CONTENT 9. Emotional Wellbeing

Profound Prosperity: Supporting the Nursery of Ripeness Within

Envision your profound scene as a rich nursery, where the seeds of trust, versatility, and taking care of oneself are planted. This section, "Close to home Prosperity," welcomes you to watch out for the nursery of your feelings, perceiving their significant effect on your ripeness process. Here, you'll investigate the specialty of developing close to home prosperity, encouraging a supporting climate where your psychological and profound states blend with your body's rhythms. Get ready to leave on an excursion that meshes profound wellbeing into the texture of your fruitfulness.

1. Embracing Feelings: Seeds of Self-Awareness

Picture feelings as seeds ready to be recognized and supported. Profound prosperity starts with embracing your sentiments, whether they're blissful, restless, confident, or questionable. By giving space to your feelings, you're recognizing your inward scene, permitting your close to home nursery to flourish.

2. Mind-Body Association: Agreement Within

Envision the brain body association as the mind boggling dance that joins your contemplations and actual prosperity. Close to home prosperity includes perceiving how stress, uneasiness, and even delight influence your chemicals and regenerative framework. By sustaining profound equilibrium, you're developing a climate that fits your internal world with your body's normal rhythms.

3. Taking care of oneself Customs: Watching out for Your Garden
Picture taking care of oneself as the sustaining contact that keeps an eye on your profound nursery. Taking part in taking care of oneself customs - whether through contemplation, journaling, or imaginative pursuits - gives comfort to your spirit. By committing time to your prosperity, you're cultivating personal versatility that turns into an establishment for richness.

4. Positive Mentality: Seeds of Hope
Envision a positive mentality as the daylight that washes your profound

nursery in warmth. Close to home prosperity includes developing contemplations that are confident, hopeful, and supporting. By sowing seeds of energy, you're establishing a climate where your psychological viewpoint lines up with the capability of origination.

5. Stress The executives: Removing Tension

Picture pressure as the weeds that take steps to eclipse your profound nursery. Profound prosperity includes rehearsing pressure the board methods, like profound breathing, care, and unwinding works out. By removing pressure, you're making a rich space where close to home equilibrium can thrive.

6. Daily reassurance: Supporting Connections

Picture everyday encouragement as the downpour that extinguishes your profound nursery's thirst. Drawing in with friends and family, support gatherings, or specialists encourages a climate where your feelings are approved and perceived. By looking for association, you're sustaining personal prosperity and making a space for recuperating discussions.

7. Resilience: Blooming In the midst of Challenges
Envision flexibility as the durable roots that anchor your close to home nursery, permitting it to face life's hardships. Close to home prosperity includes creating adapting abilities that engage you to explore difficulties with beauty. By cultivating strength, you're establishing a climate where misfortunes open doors for development.

8. Association with Accomplice: A Brought together Fruitfulness Journey

Imagine your accomplice as an individual nursery worker, keeping an eye on the close to home scene together. Profound prosperity includes open correspondence, compassion, and common help. By sharing your profound encounters, you're sustaining a bound together way to deal with richness, where your feelings interweave and prosper.

As you step into the domain of close to home prosperity, recollect that you're supporting a nursery that influences both your interior world and your ripeness process. By embracing your feelings, rehearsing, taking care of oneself, and encouraging good considerations, you're developing a climate where trust, equilibrium, and versatility flourish. This excursion is a demonstration of your profound strength, the force of care, and the profound association between close to home prosperity and ripeness.

Welcome to the reality where your profound nursery turns into a safe-haven for development, understanding, and the commitment of fresh starts.

Tending to Uneasiness and Feelings on the Ripeness Excursion: Exploring with Compassion

Envision your ripeness process as a winding way, where feelings and nerves can some of the time cast shadows out and about ahead. This section, "Tending to Tension and Feelings on the Richness Excursion," fills in as your aide through the profound scene that goes with the quest for origination. Here, you'll investigate the specialty of exploring with empathy, embracing your sentiments, and tracking down systems to oversee tension. Get ready to set out on an excursion of self-revelation, versatility, and profound prosperity as you navigate the territory of fruitfulness.

1. Embracing Feelings: Regarding Your Inward Landscape

Envision feelings as signs along your fruitfulness process, directing you toward more profound mindfulness. Tending to uneasiness and feelings starts with perceiving and embracing what you're feeling - whether it's expectation, dread, dissatisfaction, or happiness. By recognizing these feelings, you're regarding your extraordinary internal scene and making way for merciful investigation.

2. Nervousness and Richness: A Sensitive Dance

Envision nervousness as a dance accomplice on your fruitfulness process, here and there driving with vulnerability.

Tending to uneasiness includes figuring out its job and effect. It's generally expected to encounter genuine concerns during this time, however by recognizing them and looking for solid survival techniques, you're moving the equilibrium toward close to home prosperity.

3. Self-Compassion: Supporting Internal Kindness

Picture self-empathy as the sustaining demulcent that alleviates uneasiness' injuries. Tending to tension and feelings includes treating yourself with a similar delicacy you'd propose to a companion. Practice self-sympathy through good self-talk, taking care of oneself customs, and understanding that your sentiments are substantial and deserving of care.

4. Mindfulness: Mooring in the Present

Envision care as the anchor that grounds you right now. Tending to uneasiness includes rehearsing care procedures that assist you with remaining focused and oversee feelings of apprehension. By developing familiarity with your viewpoints and sensations, you're making a space where tension's hold can release.

5. Encouraging group of people: Building Extensions of Connection
Imagine your encouraging group of people as a scaffold that traverses the profound valleys of the ripeness venture. Tending to nervousness and feelings includes looking for associations with friends and family, support gatherings, or emotional wellness experts. By discussing your thoughts, you're encouraging a feeling of figuring out, sympathy, and approval.

6. Survival methods: Creating Your Toolkit

Picture survival techniques as apparatuses in your close to home tool stash, assisting you with dealing with tension's back and forth movement. Tending to tension includes tracking down methods that work for you - whether it's profound breathing activities, journaling, reflection, or participating in side interests. By outfitting yourself with survival strategies, you're enabling yourself to confront uneasiness with versatility.

7. Accomplice Correspondence: A Common Voyage

Envision your accomplice as a co-skipper on the profound journey of fruitfulness. Tending to tension and feelings includes open correspondence, permitting both of you to communicate your sentiments, fears, and expectations. By sharing this profound excursion, you're cultivating a feeling of solidarity and understanding, making a more grounded starting point for versatility.

8. Proficient Direction: Looking for Master Compassion
Imagine looking for proficient direction as enrolling a compass to explore close to home scenes. Addressing tension includes thinking about treatment or directing to investigate your sentiments and foster powerful survival methods. By looking for master direction, you're moving toward profound prosperity.

As you explore the territory of tending to tension and feelings on the richness venture, recall that you're in good company in your sentiments. By embracing feelings, rehearsing self-sympathy, and using steady methodologies, you're furnishing yourself

with devices that enable you to confront
nervousness with strength and elegance.
This excursion is a demonstration of your
solidarity, your ability for development,
and the force of exploring difficulties
with sympathy and understanding.
Welcome to the existence where tending
to uneasiness turns into a chance for
close to home recuperating,
development, and the commitment of a
more adjusted fruitfulness venture.

Building a Strong Organization: Winding around Strings of Understanding and Empathy

Envision your ripeness process as an
embroidery, woven with strings of help
that give strength and solace. This
section, "Building a Strong Organization:
Family, Companions, and Experts,"
welcomes you to embrace the force of

association as you explore the intricacies of origination. Here, you'll investigate the specialty of making a strong organization that incorporates family, companions, and experts who get it and understand your excursion. Plan to leave on an excursion of fortitude, where the bonds you fashion become a wellbeing net of grasping, support, and shared yearnings.

1. The Force of Association: Scaffolds of Understanding
Imagine association as scaffolds that range the profound holes in your richness process. Building a strong organization includes contacting the individuals who figure out your encounters, fears, and dreams. By interfacing with others who've strolled a comparative way, you're making a trap of understanding that brings comfort and fellowship.

2. Relational peculiarities: Embracing Empathetic Allies

Envision your family as a circle of empathetic partners, anxious to offer help. Building a strong organization includes conveying your requirements and feelings to friends and family. By welcoming your family into your excursion, you're cultivating an air of understanding, where compassion and support thrive.

3. Companions as Points of support: Sustaining Bonds

Picture your companions as mainstays of solidarity, offering unfaltering help as you explore your ripeness process. Building a strong organization includes trusting in companions who elevate your soul and offer in your victories and difficulties. By supporting these bonds, you're making a space where you can rest on each other with trust and credibility.

4. Accomplice Backing: A Strong
Foundation
Envision your accomplice as the
foundation of your steady organization,
remaining close by through each
diversion. Building a strong organization
includes keeping up with open
correspondence with your accomplice,
discussing your thoughts, and supporting
your association. By cultivating a unified
front, you're building up the
underpinning of your excursion together.

5. Proficient Partners: Master Guidance
Imagine experts as guides who enlighten
your way with skill and compassion.
Building a strong organization includes
looking for exhortation from ripeness
trained professionals, specialists, and
guides who have practical experience in
regenerative wellbeing. By enrolling in

their skill, you're getting an abundance of information and customized direction.

6. Support Gatherings: A Circle of Shared Experiences
Envision supports bunches as circles of shared encounters, where people meet up to elevate each other. Building a strong organization includes joining support gatherings - whether on the web or face to face - where you can interface with other people who comprehend the difficulties and triumphs of the fruitful venture. By taking part in these circles, you're tracking down approval and a feeling of having a place.

7. Online People group: Virtual Embrace
Picture online networks as virtual embraces, where close friends from around the world accumulate to offer help. Building a steady organization includes drawing in with online

discussions, virtual entertainment gatherings, and web journals committed to fruitfulness. By partaking in these spaces, you're making associations that rise above geographic limits.

8. Building Versatility: An Interweaved Journey
Envision your strong organization as strings woven into the texture of your flexibility. Building a steady organization includes recognizing that difficulties might emerge, however with the backing of friends and family and experts, you're outfitted to confront them with strength. By winding around these strings together, you're making an embroidery of trust and shared assurance.

As you leave on the excursion of building a steady organization, recall that you're encircled by people who care profoundly for your prosperity. By interfacing with family, companions, experts, and individual travelers, you're winding around a security net of grasping, compassion, and shared strength. This excursion is a demonstration of the force of human association, the bonds that inspire us, and the significant acknowledgment that you're never alone on the way to life as a parent. Welcome to the reality where fabricating a strong organization turns into a wellspring of solace, boldness, and the commitment of a local area that stands with you, through each step of your ripeness process.

CONTENT 10. Empowerment and Mindset

Strengthening and Mentality: Fashioning a Way of Solidarity and Possibility

Envision your outlook as a compass, directing your means on the excursion of fruitfulness with unfaltering assurance. This part, "Strengthening and Attitude," welcomes you to saddle the mind boggling force of your viewpoints and convictions as you explore the landscape of origination. Here, you'll investigate the craft of developing an enabled outlook that moves you forward, paying little mind to difficulties. Plan to leave on an extraordinary excursion of self-revelation, flexibility, and the acknowledgment that your mentality can shape the actual course of your fruitful journey.

1. The Force of Conviction: Molding Your Reality
Picture your convictions as the planners of your existence. Strengthening and mentality include perceiving the impact your contemplations have on your feelings, activities, and results. By developing a positive conviction framework that lines up with your richness desires, you're molding a reality where conceivable outcomes thrive.

2. Resilience: Exploring the Turns and Turns
Envision strength as the beacon that guides you through blustery waters. Strengthening and outlook include

fostering the capacity to return quickly from mishaps and difficulties. By sustaining strength, you're changing affliction into amazing open doors for development and learning on your fruitfulness process.

3. Positive Confirmations: Seeds of Empowerment
Picture positive certifications as seeds established inside the dirt of your attitude. Strengthening and mentality include utilizing certifications - positive articulations - to neutralize self-uncertainty and cynicism. By sustaining these seeds, you're developing a nursery of self-strengthening and certainty.

4. Visualization: Painting Your Ripeness Future
Envision representation as the craftsman's brush that portrays your

ideal ripeness result. Strengthening and mentality include utilizing directed symbolism to imagine achievement. By consistently picturing your process prompting origination, you're adjusting your contemplations to your profound longings.

5. Careful Appreciation: Supporting Positivity

Envision careful appreciation as the daylight that sustains your attitude. Strengthening and mentality include rehearsing appreciation for the current second and the excursion ahead. By zeroing in on the up-sides in your day to day existence, you're cultivating a climate where hopefulness and plausibility thrive.

6. Relinquishing Control: Embracing Flow

Envision relinquishing control as the demonstration of delivering the solid handle on results. Strengthening and outlook include perceiving that while you can impact your excursion, you have zero control over each viewpoint. By embracing the progression of your richness, you're permitting space for supernatural occurrences to unfurl.

7. Self-Care: An Underpinning of Strength
Picture taking care of oneself as the establishment that upholds your engaged attitude. Strengthening and mentality include sustaining your body, psyche, and soul through taking care of oneself ceremonies. By focusing on your prosperity, you're making an impression on yourself that you merit love, care, and strengthening.

8. Observing Advancement: Achievements of Growth

Envision celebrating progress as the achievements that mark your development and accomplishments. Strengthening and mentality include recognizing each step in the right direction, regardless of how little. By commending these minutes, you're building up your excursion with a feeling of achievement and inspiration.

As you set out on the excursion of strengthening and attitude, recollect that your considerations are intense devices for molding your world. By developing flexibility, positive certifications, and an engaged point of view, you're making way for a fruitful venture directed by strength and probability. This excursion is a demonstration of your ability for change, the force of your convictions, and the significant acknowledgment that your outlook can be the main thrust behind the satisfaction of your fantasies. Welcome to the reality where strengthening and mentality become the compass directing you toward a future loaded up with trust, assurance, and the commitment of a ripeness that lines up with your deepest longings.

Developing a Positive Ripeness Mentality: Supporting Seeds of Trust and Possibility

Envision your mentality as a nursery, with each thought and conviction filling in as a seed holding on to blossom. This section, "Developing a Positive Ripeness Outlook," welcomes you to step into the job of a landscaper, keeping an eye on the fruitful ground of your viewpoints and feelings as you explore your excursion to origination. Here, you'll investigate the specialty of sustaining an outlook overflowing with trust, flexibility, and steadfast faith in the chance of accomplishing your fantasies. Plan to set out on an excursion of self-revelation, strengthening, and the acknowledgment that your mentality can turn into a wellspring of inspiration and strength.

1. The Seed of Conviction: Establishing Possibilities
Imagine your convictions as the seeds that decide the idea of your fruitfulness process. Developing a positive richness outlook starts with sowing the seed of conviction - confidence in your body's ability for origination, in the way you're strolling, and in your capacity to conquer difficulties. By sustaining this seed, you're planting the establishment for an excursion enlightened by trust.

2. Strengthening in Vulnerability: Exploring with Confidence
Envision strengthening as the compass that guides you through the obscure territory of ripeness. Developing a positive ripeness mentality includes engaging yourself with information, looking for help, and stating your job as a functioning member in your excursion. By embracing strengthening, you're changing vulnerability into a chance for development.

3. Flexibility in Misfortune: Sprouting In the midst of Challenges
Picture strength as the blossom that sprouts even in the most brutal circumstances. Developing a positive ripeness mentality includes fostering the capacity to quickly return from difficulties, dissatisfactions, and snapshots of uncertainty. By supporting versatility, you're encouraging an outlook

that views difficulties as venturing stones toward your objectives.

4. Attestations of Trust: Watering the Seeds

Envision certifications as the sustaining water that takes care of your outlook garden. Developing a positive richness mentality includes utilizing positive certifications to check negative considerations. By rehashing confirmations that impact you -, for example, "My body is equipped for origination" - you're injecting your mentality with trust and energy.

5. Visualization: Arranging the Image of Success

Imagine perception as the craftsman's brush that lays out a distinctive representation of your fruitfulness achievement. Developing a positive richness mentality includes rehearsing directed symbolism where you imagine your process prompting an effective result. By drawing in your creative mind, you're adjusting your mentality to the truth you want.

6. Appreciation and Inspiration: Treating Growth

Picture appreciation as the manure that improves the dirt of your mentality garden. Developing a positive richness outlook includes embracing appreciation for your body, the help around you, and the headway you've made. By zeroing in on the thing you have, you're supporting a mentality that transmits energy.

7. Relinquishing Examination: Supporting Individual Paths

Envision relinquishing examination as the demonstration of permitting each blossom in your nursery to sprout at its own speed. Developing a positive ripeness mentality includes perceiving that everybody's process is special. By zeroing in on your own advancement and development, you're cultivating an outlook of self-empathy and tolerance.

8. Observing Each Step: Stamping Milestones
Picture festivity as the daylight that invigorates your attitude garden. Developing a positive ripeness mentality includes recognizing and commending each forward-moving step, regardless of how little. By perceiving your accomplishments, you're supporting a mentality that flourishes with progress and self-insistence.

As you set out on the excursion of developing a positive fruitfulness mentality, recollect that your contemplations have the ability to shape your world. By sowing seeds of conviction, strengthening, and versatility, and by sustaining them with certifications, perception, and appreciation, you're cultivating a nursery of energy that upholds your excursion to origination. This excursion is a demonstration of your ability for development, the force of your outlook, and the significant acknowledgment that your contemplations can be the main impetus behind the acknowledgment of your fantasies. Welcome to the existence where developing a positive fruitfulness mentality turns into an extraordinary demonstration of taking care of oneself, strengthening, and the commitment of a future sprouting with trust and plausibility.

Conquering Difficulties and Embracing Strength: The Steady Soul of Your Richness Journey

Envision your richness process as a tough way, twisting through valleys of difficulties and scaling pinnacles of assurance. This part, "Conquering Difficulties and Embracing Strength," allures you to wear the shroud of versatility as you explore the exciting bends in the road of origination's landscape. Here, you'll investigate the craft of defying difficulty with steady strength, arising out of mishaps more grounded than previously. Plan to leave on an excursion of self-revelation, strengthening, and the acknowledgment that difficulties are open doors in mask.

1. The Life structures of Difficulties: Venturing Stones to Growth
Imagine difficulties as venturing stones on your ripeness process, everyone a chance for development. Defeating difficulties and embracing flexibility

includes perceiving that misfortunes are important for the way. By survey difficulties as examples as opposed to hindrances, you're rethinking your attitude to explore them with fortitude.

2. Versatility as a Signal: Directing Through Adversity
Envision flexibility as a signal that lights your direction through the haziness of difficulties. Conquering provokes includes developing the capacity to return quickly from mishaps with determination. By embracing versatility, you're making a wellspring of solidarity that permits you to weather tempests and proceed with your excursion sincerely.

3. Attitude Change: Moving Perspectives
Picture attitude changes as the key that opens the way to strength. Conquering difficulties includes moving your point of view from "Why me?" to "What could I

learn at any point?" By reexamining difficulties as any open doors for development and self-revelation, you're engaging yourself to transcend misfortune.

4. Critical thinking Abilities: Apparatuses of Empowerment

Envision critical thinking abilities as the apparatuses that engage you to explore difficulties. Conquering difficulties includes fostering an essential way to deal with critical thinking, separating challenges into sensible advances. By cultivating critical thinking abilities, you're assuming command over your excursion and transforming difficulties into conquerable errands.

5. Self-Compassion: Embracing Imperfection

Picture self-sympathy as a delicate hug that pads your process through difficulties. Conquering difficulties includes treating yourself with thoughtfulness and figuring out, even in snapshots of trouble. By rehearsing self-sympathy, you're supporting a climate of taking care of oneself that reinforces your strength.

6. Looking for Help: Winding around a Wellbeing Net
Envision looking for help as the demonstration of winding around a wellbeing net to get you when difficulties emerge. Conquering difficulties includes connecting with friends and family, companions, experts, and care groups. By sharing your excursion and looking for direction, you're constructing an organization of understanding and sympathy.

7. Care in the Tempest: Focused In the midst of Adversity

Picture care as an anchor that keeps you grounded during difficulties. Conquering difficulties includes remaining present and drew in with your feelings, as opposed to being cleared away by them. By rehearsing care, you're cultivating close to home flexibility and remaining associated with your inward strength.

8. Observing Little Wins: Feeding Progress

Picture celebrating little wins as the sustenance that powers your process through difficulties. Beating difficulties includes recognizing even the littlest triumphs en route. By praising each step in the right direction, you're helping yourself to remember your advancement and sustaining a feeling of achievement.

As you set out on the excursion of beating difficulties and embracing versatility, recollect that your solidarity is boundless. By reviewing difficulties as any open doors for development, sustaining flexibility, and looking for help when required, you're preparing yourself to overcome impediments and rise up out of difficulty more grounded than at any other time. This excursion is a demonstration of your ability for change, the force of your soul, and the significant acknowledgment that difficulties are not barriers, but rather venturing stones on the way to your fantasies. Welcome to the existence where conquering provokes turns into a demonstration of your unyielding soul, your steady assurance, and the commitment of a future where strength makes you ready to win.

CONTENT 11. Planning for Parenthood

Making arrangements for Being a parent: Exploring the Way to Life as a parent with Planning and Purpose

Envision your excursion to life as a parent as a painstakingly diagrammed course, directed by goal and planning. This part, "Making arrangements for Being a parent," welcomes you to turn into the engineer of your family's future as you establish the groundwork for inviting another life into your reality. Here, you'll investigate the craft of fastidious preparation, smart direction, and embracing the conceivable outcomes that lie ahead. Plan to set out on an excursion of key stages, close to home status, and the acknowledgment that anticipating being a parent is an enabling demonstration that shapes the existence you're making.

1. The Outline of Life as a parent: Planning Your Path

Envision making arrangements for being a parent as portraying the outline of your family's fate. It includes assessing your status, wants, and contemplations. By planning an arrangement that lines up with your qualities and objectives, you're manufacturing a way toward the life as a parent you imagine.

2. Richness Evaluations: A Fortifying Start

Envision fruitfulness evaluations as the most important phase in planning for life as a parent. Making arrangements for life as a parent includes grasping your regenerative wellbeing through clinical assessments. By tending to any potential worries from the get-go, you're making way for a solid origination venture.

3. Monetary Status: Building a Stable Foundation

Picture monetary status as the foundation of your being a parent plan. Making arrangements for being a parent includes assessing what is going on, making a spending plan, and taking into account the expenses related with bringing up a youngster. By building a stable monetary establishment, you're guaranteeing a solid climate for your developing family.

4. Profound Arrangement: Developing Readiness

Envision close to home arrangement as supporting the dirt for being a parent's development. Making arrangements for life as a parent includes recognizing your feelings, examining assumptions with your accomplice, and embracing the progressions that accompany becoming guardians. By developing close to home preparation, you're making space for the delight, difficulties, and changes that being a parent brings.

5. Way of life Changes: Making a Family-Driven Life

Imagine how life changes as the brushstrokes paint your family-driven future. Anticipating being a parent includes adjusting your schedules, propensities, and needs to oblige your developing family's requirements. By rolling out intentional improvements, you're establishing a climate that sustains your kid's prosperity.

6. Making Emotionally supportive networks: Building a Village

Envision making emotionally supportive networks as building a town that encompasses your family with care. Anticipating life as a parent includes interfacing with companions, family, and neighborhood assets that give help, counsel, and friendship. By building an encouraging group of people, you're guaranteeing you're in good company on this groundbreaking excursion.

7. Setting up Your Home: Settling with Purpose

Picture setting up your home as the demonstration of settling, making a comfortable place of refuge for your future kid. Making arrangements for life as a parent includes setting up the nursery, coordinating basics, and childproofing your space. By guaranteeing your house is prepared, you're inviting your little one into a sustaining climate.

8. Legitimate and Pragmatic Matters: Getting Tomorrow
Picture lawful and reasonable issues as the structure that gets your family's future. Making arrangements for life as a parent includes checking on authoritative reports, like wills and guardianship arrangements, to guarantee your youngster's prosperity. By tending to these issues, you're offering your family a feeling that all is well with the world and security.

As you set out on the excursion of making arrangements for life as a parent, recollect that each step you take is a cognizant interest in your family's future. By assessing your status, tending to your wellbeing, planning genuinely and monetarily, and establishing a steady climate, you're molding the way toward life as a parent with expectation and reason. This excursion is a demonstration of your responsibility, your affection, and the significant acknowledgment that anticipating being a parent is a strong demonstration that mirrors your desires, values, and the commitment of a day to day life overflowing with delight, development, and esteemed recollections. Welcome to the reality where anticipating life as a parent turns into an extraordinary demonstration of affection, readiness, and the encapsulation of your fantasies showing signs of life.

Getting ready for Pregnancy: Exploring the Way to Being a parent with Cautious Consideration

Envision getting ready for pregnancy as establishing the groundwork for an excursion loaded up with expectation and energy. This part, "Getting ready for Pregnancy," welcomes you to leave on an excursion of cautious preparation and insightful thought as you prepare yourself for the mind blowing experience of becoming a parent. Here, you'll investigate the craft of getting ready on different fronts - monetarily, inwardly, and essentially - to guarantee a smooth change into being a parent. Plan to assemble experiences, pursue informed choices, and step into the future with a feeling of preparation and certainty.

1. Monetary Status: Building a Strong
Base

Imagine monetary availability as the
foundation of your excursion into life as a
parent. Getting ready for pregnancy
includes assessing what is happening,
making a spending plan, and anticipating
the expenses related with pregnancy,
labor, and really focusing on a child. By
building major areas of strength for an
establishment, you're making way for an
effortless excursion.

2. Profound Arrangement: Sustaining
Your Well-Being

Envision close to home readiness as
keeping an eye on the nursery of your
heart and brain. Getting ready for
pregnancy includes recognizing and
tending to any profound worries, talking
about assumptions with your accomplice,
and embracing the progressions life as a
parent brings. By supporting your close

to home prosperity, you're guaranteeing
an amicable progress into the job of a
parent.

3. Wellbeing and Health: A Consistent
Way to Parenthood
Picture wellbeing and health as the way
that makes ready for a sound pregnancy.
Planning for pregnancy includes taking
on a decent way of life, integrating
standard activity, and keeping a
nutritious eating routine. By focusing on
your prosperity, you're enhancing your
body for the excursion ahead.

4. Clinical Check-Ups: The Groundwork
of Well-Being
Envision clinical check-ups as the
mainstays of a solid pregnancy venture.
Planning for pregnancy includes booking
meetings with your medical services
supplier to address any prior ailments,
guarantee you're cutting-edge on

inoculations, and get direction on improving your richness. By looking for clinical direction, you're making a strong starting point for your pregnancy.

5. Way of life Changes: Lining up with Parenthood
Envisioning a way of life changes as the compass directs you toward being a parent. Getting ready for pregnancy includes making acclimations to your daily schedule, propensities, and needs to oblige the necessities of a developing family. By embracing these changes, you're cultivating a climate that upholds the prosperity of both you and your future kid.

6. Emotionally supportive networks: Building an Organization of Care
Envision emotionally supportive networks as the wellbeing net that gets you as you progress into life as a parent.

Planning for pregnancy includes associating with companions, family, and neighborhood assets that offer direction and help. By building an encouraging group of people, you're guaranteeing yourself a local area to rest on all through your excursion.

7. Functional Contemplations: Setting the Stage

Picture pragmatic contemplations as the stage whereupon your nurturing venture unfurls. Planning for pregnancy includes arriving at conclusions about maternity leave, childcare choices, and how to adjust work and day to day life. By tending to these useful issues, you're making a guide for a consistent change into being a parent.

8. Relationship Elements: Supporting Togetherness

Envision relationship elements as the embroidered artwork woven with the strings of organization and understanding. Planning for pregnancy includes open correspondence with your accomplice, talking about jobs and obligations, and supporting each other inwardly. By sustaining your relationship, you're making a groundwork of solidarity as you set out on this extraordinary excursion.

As you step into the domain of planning for pregnancy, recollect that every thought and choice you make adds to a smoother change into being a parent. By assessing your monetary status, sustaining your close to home prosperity, focusing on wellbeing, and making useful arrangements, you're making way for an euphoric and satisfying excursion. This is a demonstration of your commitment, your enthusiasm to embrace change, and the significant acknowledgment that getting ready for pregnancy is a caring demonstration that shapes the eventual fate of your loved ones. Welcome to the reality where planning turns into an excursion of care, strengthening, and the commitment of another section loaded up with affection, development, and treasured minutes.

Exploring the Change to Being a parent: Outlining the Course with Confidence

Envision the change to being a parent as a journey into unknown waters, loaded up with energy, challenges, and endless love. This part, "Exploring the Progress to Being a parent," welcomes you to control your boat with certainty as you set out on an excursion that changes you into a parent. Here, you'll investigate the specialty of adjusting to new jobs, embracing change, and sustaining the bonds that structure the underpinning of your developing family. Get ready to head out with astuteness, embrace the unforeseen, and explore this change with flexibility and beauty.

1. Embracing New Jobs: Molding Your Identity
Imagine the change to life as a parent as a chance to form your personality once more. Exploring this progress includes embracing the jobs of a parent, accomplice, and individual all the while. By adjusting to these jobs with an open heart, you're framing a diverse character that winds around together love, obligation, and self-improvement.

2. Evolving Elements: Fortifying Relationships

Envision changing elements as the tides that shape the connections in your day to day existence. Exploring the change to life as a parent includes discussing straightforwardly with your accomplice, acclimating to new schedules, and sustaining your association. By focusing on your relationship and establishing a strong climate, you're cultivating a bond that endures the difficulties of life as a parent.

3. Taking care of oneself in Life as a parent: Supporting Your Well-Being Picture taking care of oneself as the compass that guides you through the waters of life as a parent. Exploring this change includes setting aside a few minutes for your own prosperity in the midst of the requests of really focusing on a kid. By rehearsing and taking care of oneself, you're guaranteeing that you're

prepared to address the issues of your family with energy and imperativeness.

4. Adjusting Liabilities: Shuffling with Grace
Envision adjusting liabilities as the demonstration of watching out for numerous parts of your life. Exploring the progress to life as a parent includes tracking down harmony between nurturing, work, taking care of oneself, and connections. By overseeing liabilities with expectation and association, you're making an agreeable life that blossoms with balance.

5. Supporting Your Bond: Parent-Youngster Connection
Imagine supporting your bond as the establishment that secures your loved ones. Exploring this progress includes framing a profound association with your youngster through mindful

consideration, holding exercises, and shared encounters. By supporting this bond, you're assembling major areas of strength for the caring establishment that shapes your youngster's future.

6. Using time productively: Cruising Smoothly

Envision using time effectively as the rudder that guides your boat through the floods of life as a parent. Exploring this change includes laying out schedules, defining boundaries, and setting aside a few minutes for you as well as your friends and family. By overseeing time successfully, you're making a feeling of request and construction that upholds your family's development.

7. Looking for Help: Securing in Community

Picture looking for help as the raft that keeps you above water during difficulties.

Exploring the progress to life as a parent includes interfacing with different guardians, looking for direction, and sharing encounters. By connecting for help, you're encouraging a feeling of fellowship that advises you that you're in good company on this excursion.

8. Adaptability: Cruising through Storms Imagine versatility as the sail that gets the unavoidable trends and pushes you forward. Exploring this change includes staying adaptable and open to changes as conditions develop. By embracing versatility, you're outfitting yourself with the strength expected to weather conditions difficulties and embrace the delights of being a parent.

As you explore the change to life as a parent, recollect that you're in charge of a groundbreaking excursion. By embracing new jobs, sustaining connections, rehearsing, taking care of oneself, and encouraging areas of strength for a youngsters bond, you're controlling your boat with aim and love. This excursion is a demonstration of your capacity to embrace change, your obligation to development, and the significant acknowledgment that exploring the progress to being a parent is a groundbreaking demonstration that shapes the fate of your loved ones. Welcome to the reality where exploring this change turns into a journey of affection, association, and a truly epic commitment of shared recollections and valued minutes.

CONTENT 12.Success Stories and Inspiration

Genuine Tributes of Ripeness Wins: Stories That Enlighten the Path

Envision genuine tributes as the endearing stories of people who have arisen triumphant on their richness processes. This part, "Genuine Tributes of Richness Wins," welcomes you to step into the existences of the people who have confronted difficulties and vanquishcd them with faithful assurance. Here, you'll investigate the force of flexibility, the sorcery of trust, and the wonderful changes that unfurl when dreams work out as expected. Get ready to be charmed, enlivened, and reminded that in the midst of the preliminaries, wins anticipate.

1. Winning Over Chances: An Excursion of Resilience
Picture winning over chances as the story of opposing difficulties with faithful boldness. Genuine tributes of fruitfulness wins include accounts of people who conquered snags like fruitlessness, unnatural birth cycle, and clinical intricacies. By drenching yourself in their accounts, you're reminded that misfortunes can be venturing stones toward progress.

2. A Supernatural occurrence Called Trust: Accounts of Surprising Blessings
Envision a marvel called trust as the endearing stories of startling euphoria. Genuine tributes of ripeness wins include

records of people who had faith in the chance of being a parent despite everything. By paying attention to these accounts, you're reminded that trust has the ability to transform dreams into the real world.

3. The Strength Inside: Stories of Steadfast Determination

Picture the strength inside as the records of people who wouldn't surrender. Genuine tributes of fruitfulness wins include accounts of determined diligence, where difficulties were met with resolve. By encountering their excursions, you're motivated to develop your own internal solidarity to deal with difficulties directly.

4. Examples from the Excursion: Pearls of Wisdom

Envision examples from the excursion as the insight acquired through firsthand encounters. Genuine tributes of richness wins include experiences shared by the individuals who explored the way before you. By embracing their insight, you're furnished with direction that can shape your own choices and activities.

5. Euphoric Starting points: Stories of Delightful Starts
Envision cheerful starting points as stories that praise the delight of new life. Genuine tributes of ripeness wins include records of people who held their hotly anticipated children in their arms. By drenching yourself in these stories, you're encompassed in the delight that goes with the appearance of a loved kid.

6. From Uncertainty to Conviction: Changes Through Positivity
Envision changes through inspiration as accounts of people who transformed uncertainty into steadfast confidence. Genuine tributes of richness wins include

records of the individuals who moved
their viewpoints and supported a positive
outlook. By paying attention to their
encounters, you're roused to develop
your own confidence in the conceivable
outcomes that lie ahead.

7. Ardent Appreciation: Stories of
Fulfillment
Picture sincere appreciation as stories
that flood with appreciation for the
excursion's summit. Genuine tributes of
richness wins include records of people
who offer profound thanks for the gifts of
life as a parent. By hearing their
accounts, you're helped to embrace each
move toward remembering your own
excursion with appreciation.

8. Spreading Motivation: The Gradually
expanding influence of Triumphs
Envision spreading motivation as the
inheritance left by the people who share

their accounts. Genuine tributes of fruitfulness wins include people who decide to elevate and support others through their encounters. By accepting their motivation, you're reminded that your process can likewise influence and move the individuals who follow.

As you drench yourself in the genuine tributes of richness, recall that these accounts are a demonstration of the strength of the human soul, the influence of trust, and the extraordinary idea of steadiness. By embracing these stories, you're drawing strength from the encounters of others and tracking down consolation to confront your own difficulties earnestly. This excursion is an update that wins are individual triumphs, yet wellsprings of motivation that light the way for others to track down their own way to satisfaction. Welcome to the existence where genuine tributes become an encouraging sign, where the tales of wins become a wellspring of boldness, and where your own process will one day rouse the individuals who look for their own triumphs.

Examples of overcoming adversity and Motivation: Enlightening the Way with Win and Hope

Envision examples of overcoming adversity as reference points of light, directing your direction through the difficulties of your richness process. This part, "Examples of overcoming adversity and Motivation," welcomes you to luxuriate in the sparkle of shared wins and find motivation in the excursions of other people who have strolled the way you're on. Here, you'll investigate the force of trust, the strength of the human soul, and the resolute assurance that can transform dreams into the real world. Get ready to be propelled, inspired, and reminded that your process is essential for an embroidery woven with boldness and tirelessness.

1. The Enchantment of Trust: Directing You Forward
Picture trust as a flash that lights the fire of plausibility in your heart. Examples of overcoming adversity and motivation include embracing trust as a main impetus that drives you forward. By associating with accounts of other people who have conquered difficulties, you're arousing your own fire of conviction and assurance.

2. Win Over Difficulty: Beating the Odds
Envision wins over misfortune as a demonstration of the human soul's unstoppable nature. Examples of

overcoming adversity and motivation include gaining from the people who have confronted difficulties and arisen more grounded. By seeing others' victories, you're reminded that difficulties are not unrealistic hindrances but rather potential open doors for development.

3. Shared Excursions: Interfacing Through Experiences
Picture shared ventures as strings that weave an embroidery of aggregate encounters. Examples of overcoming adversity and motivation include associating with people who have left in comparable ways. By paying attention to their accounts, you're encouraging a feeling of kinship, knowing that you're in good company in your excursion.

4. Resolute Assurance: Fashioning Ahead

Picture enduring assurance as a power that pushes you through the hardest of times. Examples of overcoming adversity and motivation include drawing strength from the individuals who have shown exceptional determination. By seeing their diligence, you're urged to endure with your own unfaltering soul.

5. Endearing Tributes: Genuine Miracles Envision inspiring tributes as the verification that fantasies can become reality. Examples of overcoming adversity and motivation include finding out about genuine supernatural occurrences that have unfurled for other people. By drenching yourself in these stories, you're reminded that supernatural occurrences can appear in startling and lovely ways.

6. Examples from the Excursion: Intelligence Shared

Imagine illustrations from the excursion as pearls of intelligence passed down from the individuals who have strolled the way before you. Examples of overcoming adversity and motivation include gathering bits of knowledge from others' encounters. By gaining from their excursions, you're furnished with information that can illuminate your own choices and activities.

7. Defeating Questions: Energized by Positivity

Envision defeating questions as the victory of inspiration over vulnerability. Examples of overcoming adversity and motivation include seeing how others feel a little unsure into steady conviction. By submerging yourself in these accounts, you're urged to move your viewpoint and sustain a positive mentality.

8. Lighting Your Way: Enlightening the Way

Picture examples of overcoming adversity as stars that light up your way through the dimness. Examples of overcoming adversity and motivation include involving the encounters of others as directing lights. By permitting these accounts to beam on your excursion, you're embracing the insight of the people who have made ready before you.

As you drench yourself in examples of overcoming adversity and motivation, recollect that you're in good company in your excursion. By interfacing with the victories of others, you're drawing strength from their encounters and tracking down consolation to beat your own difficulties. This excursion is a demonstration of the human limit with respect to versatility, the force of shared encounters, and the significant acknowledgment that examples of overcoming adversity and motivation resemble signals that guide you toward your fantasies. Welcome to the reality where examples of overcoming adversity become a wellspring of strengthening, where the excursions of others become your directing lights, and where your own victories will one day motivate the people who emulate your example.

Rousing Excursions to Being a parent: Stories That Touch off the Fire of Possibility

Envision persuading ventures as the stories of people who have transformed their fantasies of being a parent into the real world. This section, "Inspiring

Excursions to Life as a Parent," welcomes you to step into the existences of the individuals who have dealt with difficulties directly and arose as guardians overflowing with delight and satisfaction. Here, you'll investigate the force of assurance, the flexibility of the human soul, and the groundbreaking idea of never abandoning one's fantasies. Plan to be propelled, energized, and reminded that the excursion to life as a parent is a demonstration of the steady soul that exists in all of us.

1. From Battle to Win: Revealing the Force of Resilience
Picture the excursion from battle to win as the story of overcoming deterrents with resolute assurance. Persuading excursions to life as a parent include accounts of people who resisted difficulties like barrenness, clinical difficulties, and catastrophe. By

drenching yourself in their encounters, you're reminded that strength is the foundation of achievement.

2. Touching off the Flash of Trust: Accounts of Light in Darkness
Envision lighting the flash of trust as the gladdening stories of tracking down trust amidst vulnerability. Rousing excursions to life as a parent include records of people who gripped to trust in any event, when confronted with difficulty. By engrossing these accounts, you're reminded that trust has the ability to enlighten even the haziest corners.

3. Transforming Dreams into The real world: Stories of Tenacious Pursuit
Picture transforming dreams into reality as accounts of people who never abandoned their goals. Propelling excursions to life as a parent include records of steadfast assurance, where

difficulties were met with determination. By encountering these excursions, you're propelled to seek after your fantasies with a similar determination.

4. Examples from the Way: Chunks of Wisdom
Envision illustrations from the way as the insight acquired from navigating the testing landscape. Inspiring excursions to life as a parent include bits of knowledge shared by the people who have strolled the way before you. By embracing their insight, you're enabled with information that can direct your own choices and decisions.

5. Anticipating Fresh starts: Accounts of Blissful Arrival
Envision anticipating fresh starts as stories that commend the appearance of hotly anticipated gifts. Rousing excursions to life as a parent include

accounts of people who held their valuable youngsters interestingly. By submerging yourself in these accounts, you're wrapped in the delight that accompanies satisfying a fantasy.

6. Changes Through Energy: From Uncertainty to Belief
Imagine changes through inspiration as accounts of people who transformed uncertainty into unflinching confidence. Persuading excursions to being a parent include records of the individuals who moved their viewpoints and sustained a positive outlook. By paying attention to their encounters, you're propelled to develop your own confidence in the conceivable outcomes ahead.

7. Appreciation and Satisfaction: Stories of Abundance
Picture appreciation and satisfaction as stories that flood with appreciation for

the excursion's prices. Inspiring excursions to being a parent include records of people who offer profound thanks for the endowment of life as a parent. By hearing their accounts, you're helped to relish each experience to remember your own excursion.

8. The Wave of Inspiration: Rousing Others to Act

Envision the wave of inspiration as the effect left by the people who share their accounts. Rousing excursions to being a parent include people who decide to elevate and motivate others through their encounters. By accepting their inspiration, you're reminded that your own process can likewise engage and support the individuals who look for their own ways.

As you drench yourself in the spurring excursions to life as a parent, recall that

these accounts are a demonstration of
the force of constancy, the enchantment
of trust, and the extraordinary changes
that unfurl when we won't relinquish our
fantasies. By associating with these
stories, you're saddling the strength of
shared encounters and tracking down
motivation to confront your own
difficulties with enduring assurance. This
excursion is an update that each step in
the right direction, each snag survive,
and each fantasy acknowledged is a
wellspring of inspiration that fills the fire
of opportunities for the people who hope
against hope. Welcome to the existence
where persuading ventures become a
reference point of boldness, where stories
become impetus for change, and where
your own process will one day move
others to set out on their own ways to life
as a parent.

CONTENT 13.Resources and References

Assets and References: Directing Your Way with Information and Support

Envision assets and references as the compass that guides you through your excursion to fruitfulness authority. This section, "Assets and References," welcomes you to dive into a gold mine of information, direction, and support that can enlighten your way. Here, you'll investigate an abundance of assets, from trustworthy books and sites to master guidance and steady networks. Plan to furnish yourself with data, track down comfort in shared encounters, and find the force of information as you explore your direction to richness achievement.

1. Master Direction: Exploring with Wisdom
Envision master direction as the North Star that enlightens your excursion. Assets and references offer admittance to experts who have some expertise in richness, conceptive wellbeing, and related fields. By looking for their insight, you're taking advantage of an abundance of information that can illuminate your choices and engage you with the most recent experiences.

2. Respectable Books: Pages of Wisdom
Envision trustworthy books as the libraries of intelligence you can get to. Assets and references incorporate a plenty of very much surveyed books

composed by specialists in richness, regenerative wellbeing, and nurturing. By digging into these pages, you're submerging yourself in significant data that can extend your comprehension.

3. Confided in Sites: Online Information Hubs
Picture confided in sites as the web-based archives of data and backing. Assets and references envelop sites devoted to richness, clinical direction, way of life tips, and nurturing guidance. By investigating these internet based sanctuaries, you're accessing a universe of assets readily available.

4. Steady People group: A Snare of Understanding
Picture strong networks as an organization of people who share comparative excursions. Assets and references associate you with online

gatherings, web-based entertainment gatherings, and nearby encouraging groups of people. By drawing in with these networks, you're producing associations, getting sympathy, and tracking down solace in shared encounters.

5. Clinical Establishments: Focuses of Expertise
Envision clinical foundations as signals of specific consideration. Assets and references incorporate ripeness facilities, clinical focuses, and medical clinics with experienced experts who propose particular therapies and methodology. By looking for their skill, you're entering a domain of customized answers for your special necessities.

6. Directing and Treatment: Profound Well-Being

Envision guiding and treatment as assets for supporting your close to home prosperity. Assets and references envelop emotional well-being experts who represent considerable authority in richness related concerns. By looking for their direction, you're tending to inner difficulties and developing strength all through your excursion.

7. Online courses and Studios: Learning Opportunities
Picture online courses and studios as the virtual homerooms where you can extend your insight. Assets and references offer web-based courses, studios, and classes that cover a scope of richness related subjects. By partaking in these learning open doors, you're enhancing your comprehension and range of abilities.

8. Research Studies: Science and Progress

Envision research concentrates as windows into the state of the art advancements in fruitfulness science. Assets and references remember logical investigations that shed light for new medicines, headways, and forward leaps. By staying aware of examinations, you're remaining informed about the most recent prospects.

As you submerge yourself in assets and references, recall that information is an incredible asset that can enable you to settle on informed choices, look for fitting assistance, and explore your excursion with certainty. By investigating legitimate sources, drawing in with steady networks, and looking for master direction, you're outfitting yourself with the devices expected to explore the intricacies of fruitfulness with elegance and assurance. This excursion is an update that you're in good company - a universe of data, backing, and skill stands prepared to direct you as you step into the domain of ripeness dominance. Welcome to the reality where assets and references become your partners, where information turns into your friend, and where your process is advanced by the insight and backing of the individuals who have strolled this way before you.

Clinical and Logical References: Enlightening Richness Authority with Inside and out Understanding

Envision clinical and logical references as the mainstays of information that help your mission for fruitfulness authority. This part, "Clinical and Logical References," welcomes you to dive into the profundities of exploration, studies, and master experiences that support the universe of contraceptive wellbeing.

Here, you'll investigate a large number of assets, from peer-explored articles to clinical examinations, that give a complete comprehension of the unpredictable systems overseeing fruitfulness. Get ready to arm yourself with proof based information, draw in with the bleeding edge of clinical progressions, and embrace an excursion of informed direction.

1. Peer-Inspected Articles: Experiences from MasterMinds

Imagine peer-inspected articles as the depository of shrewdness shared by clinical specialists. Clinical and logical references envelop articles distributed in respectable diaries that dive into the complexities of ripeness, regenerative science, and related subjects. By submerging yourself in these articles, you're taking advantage of the aggregate information on specialists in the field.

2. Clinical Investigations: Disentangling Ripeness Complexities

Envision clinical investigations as the research facilities where fruitfulness intricacies are unwound. Clinical and logical references envelop concentrates on led under thorough conventions that shed light on treatment adequacy, achievement rates, and state of the art mediations. By investigating these examinations, you're acquiring experiences into the results of different methodologies.

3. Research Distributions: Windows into Advancements

Picture research distributions as the windows into the most recent progressions in regenerative science. Clinical and logical references envelop distributions that feature leap forwards in fruitfulness medicines, hereditary exploration, and contraceptive advances. By staying informed concerning these distributions, you're remaining educated about the very front regarding progress.

4. Clinical Diaries: Experiences from Practitioners
Envision clinical diaries as the correspondence channels of the clinical local area. Clinical and logical references envelop diaries committed to conceptive wellbeing, fruitfulness, and obstetrics. By scrutinizing these diaries, you're taking advantage of the encounters and ability of clinical specialists who share their discoveries.

5. Master Experiences: Voices of Authority
Envision master experiences as the signal directing your way. Clinical and logical references envelop talks with digital recordings, and talks by prestigious

specialists in fruitfulness and
regenerative medication. By drawing in
with these bits of knowledge, you're
accessing the insight and experience of
pioneers in the field.

6. Scholarly Foundations: Fruitful
Reason for Knowledge
Envision scholastic foundations as the
sustaining justification for examination
and learning. Clinical and logical
references include colleges and
exploration focuses that add to ripeness
studies. By investigating their
exploration yields, you're associating
with scholarly bits of knowledge that
improve your comprehension.

7. Clinical Meetings: Exhibiting Progress
Picture clinical meetings as the features
of progress in conceptive wellbeing.
Clinical and logical references include
meetings where specialists present their

discoveries and trade thoughts. By taking part in or getting to these meeting materials, you're submerging yourself in the beat of ebb and flow research.

8. Cooperative Endeavors: Multidisciplinary Insights
Envision cooperative endeavors as the union of various fields to address richness challenges. Clinical and logical references incorporate joint investigations including hereditary qualities, endocrinology, brain science, and then some. By investigating these interdisciplinary undertakings, you're acquiring an all encompassing viewpoint on richness.

As you drench yourself in clinical and logical references, recall that proof based information enables you to go with informed choices, advocate for your prosperity, and explore the complexities of fruitful dominance. By drawing in with peer-audited articles, clinical examinations, and master bits of knowledge, you're furnishing yourself with the apparatuses to fathom the intricacies of rich science and treatment choices. This excursion is a demonstration of your devotion to grasping, your obligation to informed decisions, and the significant acknowledgment that clinical and logical references are the establishment whereupon your excursion to richness dominance is fabricated. Welcome to the reality where references become your partners, where information turns into your compass, and where your quest for ripeness dominance is enhanced by the bits of knowledge of the clinical and academic local area.

CONTENT 14. Appendices

Appendices: Your Exhaustive Tool stash for Richness Mastery

Envision indices as the mother lode of assets that go with you on your excursion to richness authority. This part, "Reference sections," is the summit of your investigation, offering a variety of instruments, formats, and helps improve your comprehension and guide your activities. Here, you'll find a different assortment of materials intended to help your undertakings, from following devices to agendas, and in the middle between. Get ready to improve your excursion with functional assets, develop your insight, and embrace an all encompassing way to deal with ripeness dominance.

1. Ripeness Following Instruments: Exploring Your Path
Envision ripeness following devices as the compass that directs your direction. Reference sections offer downloadable diagrams and layouts for observing periods, ovulation expectations, and basal internal heat level. By utilizing these apparatuses, you're furnishing yourself with information that enables your choices and activities.

2. Healthful Rules: Sustaining Your Fertility
Envision dietary rules as the recipe for feeding your contraceptive wellbeing. Informative supplements incorporate feast plans, dietary proposals, and

recipes that help richness. By observing these rules, you're advancing your healthful admission to improve your possibilities of origination.

3. Way of life Advancement Assets: Raising Your Well-Being
Picture way of life enhancement assets as outlines for making a healthy lifestyle. Informative supplements give tips to pressure the executives, work-out schedules, and rest cleanliness. By consolidating these assets, you're encouraging general prosperity that supplements your fruitfulness process.

4. Mind-Body Association Activities: Developing Internal Harmony
Picture mind-body association practices as the way to profound prosperity. Indices incorporate reflection scripts, perception activities, and methods to oversee nervousness. By participating in

these practices, you're supporting a positive mentality that adds to your ripeness achievement.

5. Clinical Experiences Glossary: Deciphering the Terminology
Envision a clinical bit of knowledge glossary as the way to grasping richness in science. Reference sections offer a glossary of terms, clarifications, and clinical ideas. By alluding to this glossary, you're exploring the language of ripeness with certainty and clearness.

6. Steady People group Registry: Interfacing with Others
Imagine a steady network catalog as the guide to tracking down close friends. Supplements list online gatherings, virtual entertainment gatherings, and neighborhood encouraging groups of people. By utilizing this registry, you're interfacing with people who share

comparative encounters and building an emotionally supportive network.

7. Fruitfulness Cordial Climate Agenda: Making Harmony

Picture a ripeness accommodating climate agenda as the manual for upgrading your environmental elements. Informative supplements incorporate tips for poison free residing, home changes, and way of life changes. By following this agenda, you're developing a climate that upholds your richness process.

8. Profound Prosperity Assets: Supporting Your Soul

Envision profound prosperity assets as the analgesic for your heart and soul. Indices give understanding proposals, online courses, and directing choices. By using these assets, you're tending to personal difficulties and encouraging versatility.

As you plunge into the reference sections, recall that these assets are intended to be reasonable, strong, and improving buddies on your excursion. By consolidating fruitfulness following instruments, nourishing rules, way of life improvement assets, from there, the sky's the limit, you're equipping yourself with a tool compartment that upgrades your endeavors. This excursion is a demonstration of your obligation to all encompassing prosperity, your commitment to informed choices, and the significant acknowledgment that informative supplements are the thorough tool compartment that prepares you to become the best at ripeness. Welcome to the reality where supplements become your guideposts, where assets become your partners, and where your quest for richness dominance is raised by the instruments and experiences readily available.

Glossary of Ripeness Terms: Translating the Language of Contraceptive Health

Envision the glossary of richness terms as your vital aspect for opening the language of contraceptive wellbeing. This segment, "Glossary of Fruitfulness Terms," is your visa to understanding the multifaceted wording that goes with your ripeness process. Here, you'll track down clarifications, definitions, and experiences into the specific language utilized by clinical experts, specialists, and the richness of the local area. Plan to explore the domain of richness with lucidity, certainty, and a developed comprehension of the ideas that shape your way.

1. Fertility: The capacity to consider and bear youngsters, demonstrating the contraceptive capability of an individual or a couple.

2. Ovulation: The arrival of a full grown egg from the ovary, normally happening mid-cycle, which is urgent for origination.

3. Feminine Cycle: The normal grouping of hormonal changes that prompts ovulation and, on the off chance that not prepared, period.

4. Basal Internal heat level (BBT): The body's most minimal temperature is still, frequently estimated after waking, which can demonstrate the ripe window.

5. Ovulation Indicator Units (OPKs): Tests that identify chemical levels to foresee when ovulation is probably going to happen.

6. Infertility: The failure to imagine following an extended time of unprotected intercourse, or a half year for ladies north of 35.

7. Helped Regenerative Innovations (ART): Operations that help with origination, remembering for vitro treatment (IVF), intrauterine insemination (IUI), and the sky's the limit from there.

8. In Vitro Preparation (IVF): A strategy where an egg is treated external to the body and the subsequent incipient organism is embedded into the uterus.

9. Intrauterine Insemination (IUI): A methodology where sperm is set straightforwardly into the uterus to expand the possibilities of treatment.

10. Undeveloped organism Transfer: Setting a treated incipient organism into the uterus during an IVF cycle.

11. Gamete: A developed conceptive cell (sperm or egg) that can join with one more gamete to frame a zygote.

12. Zygote: The cell shaped by the combination of sperm and egg, which in the end forms into an undeveloped organism.

13. Endometrium: The coating of the uterus that thickens during the period and gives a supporting climate to an undeveloped organism.

14. Fallopian Tubes: Tubes that transport the egg from the ovaries to the uterus, where preparation ordinarily happens.

15. Insemination: The presentation of sperm into the female regenerative plot, either normally or through helped contraceptive methods.

16. Fertilization: The association of a sperm cell with an egg cell, bringing about the development of a zygote.

17. Gonadotropins: Chemicals that invigorate the ovaries to create eggs and direct the monthly cycle.

18. FSH (Follicle-Invigorating Hormone): A chemical that advances the development of ovarian follicles and invigorates the creation of eggs.

19. LH (Luteinizing Hormone): A chemical that triggers ovulation and the arrival of an egg from the ovary.

20. Sperm Count: The convergence of sperm in a given volume of semen, an element that influences male fruitfulness.

Exploring the glossary of ripeness terms enables you to discuss actually with clinical experts, grasp conversations inside the richness local area, and settle on informed conclusions about your contraceptive wellbeing. By getting to know these definitions, you're entering the universe of richness with a recently discovered clearness, guaranteeing that you're prepared to decipher clinical conversations, grasp methodology, and promoter for your prosperity. This excursion is a demonstration of your obligation to learning, your devotion to understanding, and the significant acknowledgment that the glossary of richness terms is your compass in the unpredictable scene of contraceptive wellbeing. Welcome to the existence where phrasing turns into an extension to information, where definitions become your partners, and where your quest for fruitful dominance is improved by the language that characterizes your excursion.

Fruitfulness Supporting Recipes and Dinner Plans: Sustaining Your Way to Parenthood

Envision richness helping recipes and feast plans as the culinary guide that upholds your excursion to being a parent. This part is committed to furnishing you with delectable and supplement rich dinners intended to improve your regenerative wellbeing. Here, you'll find an assortment of recipes and feast designs that are nicely created to give the fundamental supplements, nutrients, and minerals your body needs to upgrade fruitfulness. Plan to relish seasons that sustain your prosperity, develop hormonal equilibrium, and establish the groundwork for your ripeness achievement.

1. Prolific Establishments Breakfast: Empower Your Day
Begin your morning with a decent breakfast that incorporates complex carbs, lean proteins, and solid fats. A bowl of oats finished off with new berries and a sprinkle of chia seeds gives fiber, cell reinforcements, and omega-3 unsaturated fats that help hormonal equilibrium.

2. Green Goddess Smoothie: A Supplement Stuffed Delight

Mix an invigorating smoothie with spinach, avocado, banana, and almond milk. This green creation is plentiful in folate, potassium, and vitamin E, all of which add to conceptual wellbeing and in general prosperity.

3. Mediterranean-Propelled Lunch: Energetic and Satisfying

Partake in a Mediterranean-motivated lunch with a quinoa salad highlighting beautiful chime peppers, cucumbers, cherry tomatoes, and feta cheddar. Sprinkle with olive oil and lemon juice for solid fats and an eruption of flavor.

4. Omega-3 Rich Supper: Salmon Sensation

Enjoy a supper that incorporates barbecued salmon prepared with spices and a side of steamed broccoli. Salmon is an extraordinary wellspring of omega-3 unsaturated fats, which assume a part in directing chemicals and supporting richness.

5. Plant-Based Power Bite: Feeding Energy

Nibble on a small bunch of blended nuts and seeds for a portion of plant-based protein, sound fats, and zinc. Zinc is known to help contraceptive wellbeing and lift safe capability.

6. Bright Vegetable Sautéed food: Nutrients Galore

Set up a vegetable pan fried food with a rainbow of ringer peppers, carrots, snow peas, and tofu. This dish is loaded with cancer prevention agents, nutrients, and minerals that add to general wellbeing.

7. Berry Happiness Treat: Sweet and Nourishing

Enjoy a treat that joins Greek yogurt with a variety of new berries. Berries are plentiful in cell reinforcements, fiber, and nutrients that advance regenerative wellbeing.

8. Hydration with Natural Teas: A Taste of Wellness

Remain hydrated with natural teas like chamomile, vex, and red raspberry leaf. These teas are known for their likely advantages in supporting hormonal equilibrium and regenerative wellbeing.

9. Adjusted Dinner Plans: Seven days of Supplement Rich Delights

Follow a fair feast plan that incorporates different supplement thick food varieties. Consolidate entire grains, lean proteins, solid fats, and a wealth of foods grown from the ground to make dinners that help richness and in general prosperity.

10. Careful Eating Practices: Supporting Body and Soul
Integrate careful eating rehearses into your everyday practice, relishing each chomp and valuing the sustenance it brings. Developing a positive relationship with food can decidedly influence your general wellbeing and richness venture.

By embracing these richness supporting recipes and feast plans, you're feeding your body with the supplements it requires to flourish. Each dish is a demonstration of your obligation to comprehensive prosperity, your commitment to pursuing informed decisions, and the significant acknowledgment that the food sources you eat assume an imperative part in forming your richness process. Welcome to the reality where flavors become partners, where sustenance becomes strengthened, and where your quest for fruitful dominance is improved by the culinary enjoyments that help your way to life as a parent.

CONCLUSION

"Ripeness Authority Guide: Exploring Your Way to Parenthood"

Leaving on the excursion to life as a parent is a groundbreaking encounter that requires information, devotion, and an exhaustive methodology. The "Fruitfulness Dominance Guide" is your priceless sidekick through this unpredictable way, offering an all encompassing investigation of all features connected with richness, regenerative wellbeing, and the quest for life as a parent. From grasping the intricacies of fruitfulness to embracing a sustaining way of life, from deciphering the study of generation to looking for master exhortation, this guide investigates every possibility.

Opening Knowledge: Start by unwinding the complexities of fruitfulness, directed by master bits of knowledge and a glossary that interprets particular phrasing. Draw in with the clinical and logical references that support your figuring out, empowering you to settle on educated decisions each step regarding the way.

Supporting Great Being: Raise your prosperity through nourishment, way of life streamlining, and stress the board strategies that fit the psyche and body. Investigate richness supporting recipes and dinner designs that give the fundamental supplements to improve your regenerative wellbeing.

Science and Expertise: Dig into the study of generation, uncovering the intriguing cycles that lead to origination. Submerge yourself in clinical bits of knowledge, from helped regenerative advancements to figuring out hormonal equilibrium, engaging you to explore the clinical scene with certainty.

Mind-Body Connection: Develops the strong brain body association, outfitting the capability of contemplation, perception, and profound prosperity rehearses. Figure out how a positive mentality can shape your excursion and improve your rich dominance.

Support and Empowerment: Fabricate a strong organization that incorporates family, companions, experts, and online networks. Investigate persuading examples of overcoming adversity that rouse you to conquer difficulties, showing the victory of assurance and strength.

Groundwork for Parenthood: As you approach the edge of life as a parent, outfit yourself with monetary, profound, and commonsense contemplations. Explore the progress to life as a parent, recognizing the progressions and difficulties that lie ahead.

Embrace Resilience: Embrace difficulties with versatility, tracking down strength in misfortunes and exemplifying the engaging mentality expected to vanquish hindrances. Develop the positive fruitfulness mentality that makes you ready for progress.

The "Fruitfulness Dominance Guide" is in excess of a manual — a complete asset changes your excursion into a deliberate journey for ripeness dominance. With master direction, steady assets, and an abundance of information, you're engaged to explore the intricacies of fruitfulness with certainty and lucidity. This guide is a tribute to your assurance, your quest for comprehensive prosperity, and your faithful obligation to understanding your fantasy of life as a parent. Welcome to an existence where information, backing, and strengthening join to enlighten your way to ripeness dominance.

Finishing up Your Fruitfulness Authority Excursion: Embracing Trust and Empowerment

As we draw the last pages of the "Fruitfulness Dominance Guide," it's a snapshot of reflection and expectation. The excursion you've set out upon, from the absolute first section to the last, has been a demonstration of your steady obligation to figuring out, developing, and strengthening. You've dug into the intricacies of richness, developed a feeding way of life, bridled the influence of science and skill, and supported the indispensable brain body association that shapes your way.

In these pages, you've experienced the narratives of the people who have prevailed over difficulties, the direction of specialists who enlighten the way ahead, and the assets that engage you to go with informed decisions. You've investigated the profundities of your own strength, perceiving that mishaps are simply venturing stones on the way to life as a parent.

As you stand at the cusp of probability, recall that this excursion isn't just about the objective — it's about the change you've gone through. You've filled in figuring out, produced associations with a local area of help, and sharpened the mentality that moves you forward. Your quest for rich dominance is a demonstration of your solidarity, your soul, and your readiness to embrace the unexplored world.

With the information you've acquired, the assets you've gotten, and the strengthening you've developed, you're ready to push ahead with trust and certainty. The street ahead may in any case hold difficulties, however furnished with shrewdness and braced by the excursion you've attempted, you're outfitted to confront them with strength and elegance.

May this guide keep on filling in as a wellspring of motivation, direction, and support as you explore the way to life as a parent. As you turn the last page, realize that your quest for fruitfulness dominance is an excursion that rises above these words. It's an excursion of the heart, an excursion of strengthening, and an excursion that is particularly yours.

Embrace the expectation that energizes your fantasies, commend the strength that impels your undertakings, and recall that your process is a demonstration of your mental fortitude and assurance. Welcome to the section of your life where fruitful dominance turns into a reality, and where the ability to shape your future lies immovably in your grasp.